A PROMISE TO REM[...]
THE NAMES PROJECT
BOOK OF
LETTERS

edited by JOE BROWN

AVON BOOKS ◆ NEW YORK

A PROMISE TO REMEMBER: THE NAMES PROJECT BOOK OF LETTERS is an original publication of Avon Books. This work has never before appeared in book form. All letters in this book are being published with the permission of the letter writers.

AVON BOOKS
A division of
The Hearst Corporation
1350 Avenue of the Americas
New York, New York 10019

Copyright © 1992 by The NAMES Project
Cover photograph by Tom Alleman, courtesy of The NAMES Project
Panel photographs by Alain McLaughlin
Published by arrangement with The NAMES Project
Library of Congress Catalog Card Number: 91-26420
ISBN: 0-380-76711-2

Library of Congress Cataloging in Publication Data:

A Promise to remember: the names project book of letters / edited by
  Joe Brown.
      p.   cm.
     1. AIDS (Disease)—Patients—United States—Biography. 2. NAMES
Project AIDS Memorial Quilt. 3. Quiltmakers—United States—
Correspondence.   I. Brown, Joe, 1958–
RC607.A26P77   1991
362.1′969792′00922—dc20   91-26420
[B]   CIP

First Avon Books Trade Printing: August 1992

AVON TRADEMARK REG. U.S. PAT. OFF. AND IN OTHER COUNTRIES, MARCA REGIS-TRADA, HECHO EN U.S.A.

Printed in the U.S.A.

OPM   10 9 8 7 6 5 4 3 2 1

This book of letters is dedicated to Scott Lago, who dedicated his life to stitching the Quilt together, and to making sure people everywhere could see it and understand.

*

The editor is grateful to David Lemos, Geoffrey Woolley and Danny Sauro, whose love, belief and support made this book possible.

My thanks also to Mary and Joseph Brown, Carolyn and Steven Reidy, David Highfill and Marv Jensen. In San Francisco, many thanks for help and hospitality to Lee Fitzgerald, Brian Johnson and Ken Stevens, and, at the NAMES Project, to Cindy "Gert" McMullin, Sandy O'Rourke, Eric Hallquist, Marcel Miranda III, Michele Cinq Mars, Lance Henderson, Scott Osten, Andy Ilves, Danny Linden, Art Gaudet and Cindy Ruskin. In Washington, D.C., thanks to *The Washington Post*, Don Brazeal, Jeanne Cooper, Bruce Lederer, Mireille Key, Bob Kirsh, Jay Watkins, Jeanette Buck, Doug Favero, Carolyn Swift, Kara Swisher, Janet Duckworth, Amy Ziff and Jay Slot.

And thanks especially to Rich Adler, for love and encouragement beyond words.

*

A special note of appreciation to all the letter writers, and the members of the NAMES Project chapters throughout the country.

Editor's Note:

Due to the fear and prejudice that still exist in our society, some contributors have requested that their letters remain unsigned. These letters are denoted by a spool symbol.

Even the death of friends will inspire us as much as their lives . . .

Their memories will be encrusted over with sublime and pleasing thoughts, as monuments of other men are overgrown with moss; for our friends have no placc in the graveyard.

—HENRY DAVID THOREAU

INTRODUCTION

One spring day in 1987, a group of strangers met in San Francisco's Castro district to discuss a new idea. Although from different backgrounds, each had been touched in some way by the AIDS epidemic and each had made a personal commitment to help stop this disease.

The idea was the Quilt: a fabric patchwork bearing the names of people lost to AIDS; men, women and children remembered by their families and loved ones with 3' by 6' cloth panels.

We wanted to illustrate the enormity of the AIDS crisis by revealing something of the lives behind the statistics, to provide evidence of the calamity that we saw unfolding. We wanted to reach out to all the different kinds of people whose lives had been invaded by AIDS so that they could be strengthened in their personal struggles. And we wanted to give the world a powerful symbol of compassion and unity, an example of how we expected people everywhere to respond to this terrible challenge.

We chose the symbol of the Quilt in a deliberate effort to evoke and recapture the traditional American values that had yet to be applied to this apparently "nontraditional" situation—values of cooperation, mutual respect and individual freedom.

And we began to sew. Word spread slowly at first but gradually the panels we had sewn for our friends were joined with the names of many others. By late summer, new Quilt panels were arriving in our workshop every day. The Quilt was displayed for the first time on October 11, 1987 on the Capitol Mall in Washington, D.C. It contained 1,920 panels, most sewn with the names of young gay men.

By the time we returned to San Francisco, our mailbox was overflowing with letters from cities and towns all over the United States. In each envelope we found the same request: "Please, bring the Quilt to our town." So we bought a truck and set out on the first of what would be many tours, visiting the twenty largest U.S. cities. The Quilt grew as we traveled, for in every city we were presented with scores of new panels.

By October 1988, when the Quilt was displayed for the second time in our nation's capital, it had grown to include 8,288 panels. By 1989, the Quilt contained 11,000 panels when we journeyed again to Washington, D.C.

As the epidemic has grown and changed, so has the Quilt grown and changed. The early names, those of young gay men, have been joined by ever-increasing numbers of women and children. Every year we sew into the Quilt more panels for African-Americans, Hispanics, Asians and Native Americans— more Quilts made by parents for their children, more Quilts made by children for their parents.

We have also brought the Quilt to 30 nations around the world, helping people on every continent understand the AIDS epidemic in its true global context. As we have traveled with the Quilt across the United States and around the world, we have found— everywhere we go—that ordinary men, women and children do understand, do know what must be done. For them there is no mystery, no cause for controversy or debate: the sick are to be cared for; the dying are to be comforted; and the full resources available to our society must be employed to educate our people and find a cure.

We believe that our country today possesses the institutions and knowledge necessary to eradicate AIDS. As a nation, we have had to struggle not only against a virus, but against parallel epidemics of apathy, misinformation and outright bigotry. The NAMES Project is not a political organization; we take no position on the various legislative and policy issues surrounding the epidemic. From its inception, however, the NAMES Project has sought to impact the political process by helping our leaders and citizens find the will to win.

As the AIDS Memorial Quilt enters its sixth year, I would like to express my deep gratitude to the women and men of the NAMES Project, the staff, volunteers and, especially, the panelmakers. Their letters, sent to us with their Quilts, make up this book. Woven together, they tell a story of great pain and rage, love and courage. They were written for you as the Quilt was created: with hope that you would be moved—moved to act.

Cleve Jones
Founder
The NAMES Project
June, 1992

I'll never forget seeing the Quilt for the first time.

I was one of the half-million men, women and children who gathered on the green grass of the Mall for the National Gay and Lesbian March on Washington in October 1987. Out of curiosity, I decided to walk over and have a look at this "giant quilt for AIDS" that had been unfurled that autumn morning.

I meandered among the hundreds of colorful panels, impressed and quietly moved by the scope and originality of the memorial. Then I happened upon a panel made by a child for her older brother, a stranger to me, and was moved to tears. My friends had to lead me away.

It was the first time I had been able to cry for friends lost, for friends I feared I would someday lose, for myself. For all of us.

Come to think of it, it was the first time I had cried in years. I'm grateful for that healing moment.

In the four years since, I've seen the Quilt do its essential work many times. A decade into the AIDS epidemic, the Quilt has visited our nation's capital four times, and continues to take its message of compassion and consolation around the country and the world, providing adults and children a way to talk about AIDS, loss and love.

For those who have lost someone they loved, the Quilt is a place to put the memories, and a place to do something in the face of an awful helplessness. It touches the suffering, the bereaved, the fearful. And it touches those who had previously felt unaffected by AIDS.

No one leaves the Quilt unmoved.

Each panelmaker contributing to the Quilt is asked to write a letter about the person they are remembering. These letters—there are nearly 14,000 of them in The NAMES Project archives at the San Francisco workshop—are astonishingly diverse and potent, as colorful and idiosyncratic as the quilts themselves.

Written by parents, partners and caregivers, the letters tell the story behind the quilt panels. Poetic, dramatic, sometimes melodramatic, always real and felt, full of the small moments and gestures that are the stuff of life, they crystallize a personality, often so vividly and compactly that any short story writer would be proud to claim them as his own.

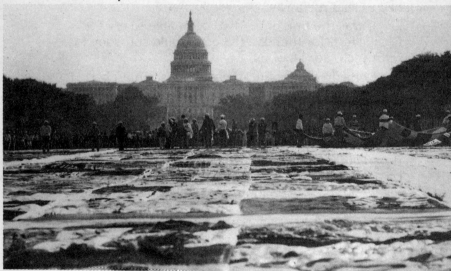

But so often the writers want and need to tell their own story, as well. In caring for a person in extremis, they have been called to do something they never would have anticipated.

And in sharing their grief in fabric and in words, they speak of how they have been enlarged, finding strength and eloquence they never knew they had.

As each quilt panel is created with the knowledge that someone will see it and share the memory, each letter is written in hope that someone, someday will read it. Some letters speak directly to the loved one, sharing feelings there was never time or words for in this life. Some speak to an "ideal reader," as if in a private diary, musing on the big questions of life and love and death and beyond.

Again and again, the letter writers tell us, "I am changed" . . . "My life will never be the same." Their definition of what it is to be a lover, mother, brother, friend is larger now. If there's a lesson to be learned from AIDS, it's here.

As I read these letters at The NAMES Project workshop, I was in awe of these people, as writers, as lovers, as fearful and brave human beings. They have so much to share. And they want to share with their readers the people they have loved.

Letter writing is an intimate form of communication. Some say it is a lost art. But it is truly living here. You can come back to the images, emotions and memories captured in a letter again and again.

What you do not see in this book is the personal touch: the handwriting, painstaking and formal, or pained and shaky; the stationery, childlike or elegant; the photos and mementos people included in keeping their promise to remember.

Authors, poets, playwrights, screenwriters, dancers, and painters have documented and dramatized the effects and emotions surrounding the AIDS crisis. Historians, politicians and medical analysts continue to examine these issues in print and on podiums.

But these letters are the real, raw, unprocessed stuff of life with AIDS. And like the individual lives they speak of, the letters cannot be forced into a category or chapter or chronology.

A Promise to Remember is a Quilt in words. The people in it live on in memory side by side, a testimony to the complexity and variety of people affected by AIDS. And to the patience and infinite expression of human love and compassion.

Certainly no book can recreate the awesome hush, the color and power that is the physical experience of the Quilt. But if you wander through this book of letters as if through the aisles of the Quilt, they may answer some questions.

They may express something you have been searching your soul to say.

They may comfort and console you.

They may make you laugh. They will certainly make you cry.

They may move you to anger, and then to action.

Each letter demands attention and time.

"After all," asks one of these letters, remembering a man named Raymond, "isn't that what each of us wants? Not to be leveled into facelessness but to be treated as a unique, inimitable person?"

Always remember,

Joe Brown

February 1992

Dear NAMES Project:

I stood before the NAMES and did not see a monument to gloating death.

I saw a measureless garden of imperishable, multicolored blossoms.

I saw a richly textured, seamless fabric, a living tapestry uniting friends, lovers, families, with handiwork proclaiming undiminished love, commitment and dedication.

I saw survivors weeping, embracing, scattering flowers upon finely embroidered affirmations to conquer this epidemic, vanquish bigotry, overcome ignorance—and the sermon the NAMES Project is preaching held me in its grip and overwhelmed me.

Only by healing can we be healed.
Only by loving can we be loved.
Only by caring can we be cared for.
Only by reaching out can we be touched . . .

Stephen Wolf

July 21, 1988

Dear God,

Please take the bits and pieces that make up the fabric of my life and use them for your purpose. Build a definite pattern so that those about can be sure of a "comforting" nature. May the light and dark parts mesh their beauty to reflect your love.

Please give the backing of my quilt the firmness to hold secure and immovable my innermost beliefs and my love for you. May my backing be flexible enough to see other points of view and to look for good in all I meet. Help me to see that my imperfections and shortcomings are things on which I can improve, but only you are perfect—that you love me in spite of my faults.

Heavenly Father, help this quilt to have a life of service, so that when life is over, the comfort, sacrifices and lessons learned will live on in those lives it has touched. Amen.

Mary Esther Carter,
Anderson, Indiana

To Whom It May Concern:

I was wondering if you would be kind enough to give or rather send me information on making a quilt. What's the best or whatever is the right material to use and also the right size and whatever else I should know how to make one. And also where to send it, when it's made.

You see this was the one thing in my life I was not looking forward to. But it has come to pass, and I'm so full of grief over the loss of my beloved son Vito Russo. He passed away this past November 7th (how I hate that day). My life will never be the same without him. I'm sure you have seen him on the documentary "Common Threads"—the story of the quilts.

My beautiful, always smiling, loving son whom I adored is gone and I'm so heartbroken over losing him. Please forgive me for getting carried away. I did not mean to do that, forgive me . . .

Vito has often spoken of the wonderful work you people have done. What a sad job to have. I pray God someday it will all be put to rest forever.

God bless—and many thanks for whatever help you can give me.

Sincerely,
Annie Russo

How does a mother go about creating a memorial to her son by representing his life on a 3′ × 6′ piece of cloth?

This was the question I asked myself over and over again, after I decided to honor my son Mike by creating a panel in his memory for the NAMES Project Quilt.

As I began to design Mike's panel and lay out the pieces, I felt as though it was the saddest and most beautiful experience of my life—somehow merging the pain of burying my son in October of 1986 with the joy of giving birth to him 37 years ago.

Then, when I took the pieces to my daughter-in-law's house to sew them together (she has a sewing machine) I knew that this experience—creating the panel—truly became an all-family project.

And I knew it was a joint family effort that would have pleased Mike very much . . .

. . . all across America there are other mothers like me, as well as fathers, grandparents, sisters, brothers, sons, daughters, nieces, nephews, lovers and friends, who have found themselves—or soon will—drawn to the Quilt by the immense power of its hope and humanity . . .

I did it for two reasons—for Mike and for all the others who've been lost to AIDS, and for myself and all the others who've lost them.

Sue Caves

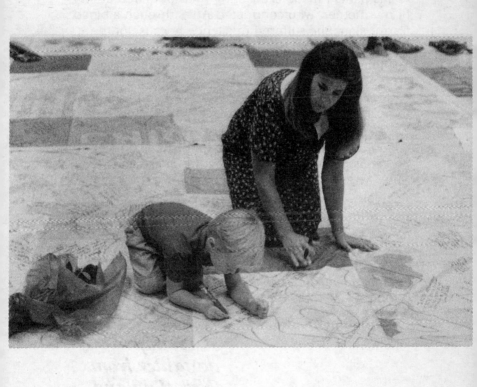

This panel I made is a lasting memorial in memory of my mother, who contracted AIDS through a blood transfusion. She suffered in silence because of the social stigma of AIDS.

Please don't make these victims embarrassed and ashamed of their illness, but reach out in love and embrace them. When we begin to love, we can begin to heal one another.

My mother loved the ocean, palm trees and her beautiful flower garden. I have faith she is now in a gorgeous garden surrounded by the peace and love of God.

You were very brave, Mom, and it hurt me to see you suffer. You were a wonderful mother who taught me so much about life. I love you and I miss you, Mom.

I pray that people will become more compassionate and understanding of the tremendous hurt and loneliness these people and their families endure.

A loving
daughter from
New England

I thought about this panel for a long time before I started it. Steve had left a note listing three things that he would like to have on it—his dogs, the faces of the theatre, and a rose. I've never seen a panel, only pictures, but I am sure they all developed as this one did. I wanted it to express humor, thoughtfulness, and above all, love—a condensed version of Steve's life.

We loved him very much.

*Norman and
Olive Anderson
(mom and dad)*

For anyone who knew him it would take volumes, not one or two pages, to do him justice. Bright, handsome, giving, caring, loving, fair, and humorous. Very humorous. Always a friend to any that needed one. God really loves me! He gave me this wonderful person for 11 years. By my wish, I confess, not long enough . . .

Making this panel has not been easy. I am by far not the only one who has done so or knows how painful it is to do it. It is not perfect, and I have cried about that. But J.T. is happy with it anyway, I know. If I could make it as glorious as this love I have in my heart for this man, it would blind all who gaze upon it.

I still love and miss my best buddy.

Love to all who should ever read this.

Brent Fleek

October 6, 1990

When you told me you had AIDS, so long ago in 1983, I hugged you. And that was the only time I remember seeing you cry. No one would touch you anymore, you said. Your friends had become afraid and could not hold you close . . .

You know, don't you, that I will do my best to see that no one with AIDS will have to live without love and hugs . . .

Joe was one of the early victims.

We lost a loving man to something they had only just begun to call "AIDS."

We met in our prime and spent our youth together. What a shame he wasn't allowed to grow old.

Joe loved to draw. This banner is made from an early drawing he did, called "Dawn."

Dear God, let it symbolize a new dawn free from AIDS.

Amen.

Mikel Ambrose

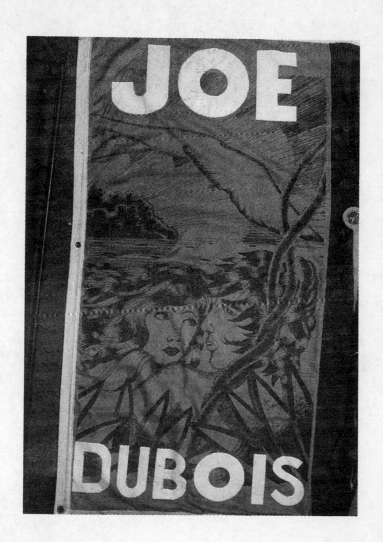

The feelings that have gone into making this panel have been overwhelming. I am not able to attach words to accompany the panel. This is the third time I am rewriting what I have written.

Harry and I were in high school together in a small town in Pennsylvania. He was one year behind me. One afternoon, when I was very depressed, he listened and helped. We didn't know each other too much more than that.

I learned he grew up and became a psychologist and moved to Texas. I became a social worker and moved to California. And one day, 20 years after high school, I learned he died of AIDS.

The colors (blue and yellow), Star of David, and numbers (tattoo) on the panel are meant to awaken memories of the other 20th century Holocaust and the many who watched without protest. Thank you for giving me a place to put my feelings. Thank you for giving all of us a way and a place to mourn and remember.

Bernie Barzal

... I have known so many good friends who have died of AIDS I could not consider making it for just one friend, so I decided to make my panel in memory of all of them . . .

I chose to include my name on the panel, not because I feel I am dying of AIDS but because I have AIDS and know all about the pain and suffering of AIDS. I have been hospitalized four times, three times with pneumocystis pneumonia. I know what it is like to be shunned by nurses and friends, hospital employees refusing to come into your room and when they did, they were covered in plastic gloves and smocks. When your meals were placed outside your room outside your door because no one would bring the food into your room . . .

I am lucky that I have wonderful loving friends who have supported me throughout this ordeal and are the reason I am alive today.

I know I am not the world's greatest seamstress, but it was all done by hand and I spent many hours on it. Every stitch was a labor of love.

If just one person is touched enough by it to try to understand what living with AIDS is like or to help someone with AIDS or by donating money or time to research or helping victims of this ugly disease, then every stitch was worth it in their memory.

Michael Paul

May 26, 1988

RICHARD ARLEN KIRKMAN, JR. ═══════

Today is October 6, 1989. I am sitting on a park bench watching volunteers set up the NAMES Project Quilt. It keeps sprinkling off and on. I feel the drops and imagine them as tears shed and to be shed.

My brother, Kirk, died of AIDS complications on July 9th of this year. He had tested positive two years ago. He lost his dear friend, John, in January of this year. Now they are together.

He would call me at all hours to chat or cry, mostly to dream! Recently he moved from San Francisco to Naples, Florida. He wanted to be closer to his family. He found an apartment condo to rent. Bought beautiful furniture and art. He was ready to settle down and have a real home all of his own.

After three days in his new home he had trouble breathing so he went to the hospital. What he thought was allergies was in fact "pneumonia." I learned to hate that word. After two days he was not responding to treatment and was put on a respirator. For 21 long days he struggled till a quiet end.

Talking and laughing were his loves. The worst for me was not hearing his voice those last days. He wrote pages of notes, but no sound. Actually at one point I was forbidden to be funny and sarcastic because he couldn't laugh.

Such pain he had endured standing by his friends. He had decided not to tell us he had tested positive. I point-blank asked. I was the only family member who knew. "The Plan" was that his lawyer would contact me after his death. When he was admitted to the hospital he called me. His last spoken words to me, "Mona, I love you, 'The Plan' is off, I am scared."

Of course, I was on the next plane. My parents arrived first, then I and then my sister with her baby. Kirk had never seen the baby. He was glad we were there. If love could cure!

Each day he slowly could not breathe. As I sat clutching his hand, watching his heartbeat get slower and slower, I felt a joy, strangely enough. He had once told me he had lived by his own rules and tunes. Everything he had ever wanted to do he had done except two. He never had a child and he never went to Europe, but he had his ticket. In fact, he would be there now.

Kirk was the only person in all my life that accepted me for me. Never asking for anything more or anything less of me. The simple things were his joy. Walking on a beach from sunrise to sunset. Being outdoors with the "Colors of the World."

My brother was a source of strength and power to me. I love him. His life still lives with my every breath because he is part of my soul and I his. This letter has helped me. Maybe it will help someone else one day. There are so many things in life to enjoy. One simple one is a memory. My memories are strong for you, Kirk, and I never part or replace a single one. Remember this one. The most special one!

With loving memories,
your sister,

Ramona Goodrich

JOHNNIE F. HERD

My son, Johnnie F. Herd, was a very special person, not only to his family, but to all who knew him. He brought joy to all. He cared for many boys and a baby whose parents had disowned them. He worked when he was very ill to buy food for those who needed it.

He was a professional horse trainer most of his life. He also gave equestrian lessons to young people who won many awards on the national level. Johnnie won the Appaloosa World Championship in 1979 and 1981. He quit training in 1985 and made barbering his work. He was wonderful in this field also. He made many dear friends and sure helped a lot of people's looks. All kidding aside, he was special.

He became ill in July 1985. He was on many testing programs for different drugs. AZT helped for two-and-one-half years. On September 6, 1989, Johnnie's life ended. He said he was excited to be going home to God.

He was our special ray of sunshine, and we are lost without him.

Thank you for the wonderful work you are doing in the displaying of the quilt panels. Our prayers are that through God's intervention something will be developed that will kill this killer virus.

I am a mother who loved unconditionally, and I was taught how to live and how to die with dignity by my son. My only son.

Patsy R. Herd

Dear Goober,

I can't do it. I've tried, but I can't make your panel yet. It's ironic, isn't it? After we've both had so much experience with the NAMES Project; helped so many other people to remember, get angry, grieve, and begin to let go by creating memorial panels to add to the Quilt.

We were there in the beginning, preparing for the inaugural display and sewing Doug's panel. Remember traveling that first year with the Quilt? The 1987 display in Washington was so exciting, so incredibly sad and cathartic, yet so hopeful.

It was four years ago today—at dawn—when the Quilt was unfolded for the first time. We both read names. What a powerful feeling to speak those names and to hear them reverberate over the National Mall toward the Capitol. You read Doug's name, then we sobbed in each other's arms as the sun rose over the city.

Then came the first national tour—the New York display with my family; Seattle and Portland with your family. They all came, and they also came around. The Quilt helped them to understand what it was we were going through. Then we were back in Washington again that October—1988. You on "Nightline"—such a great spokesperson for the cause—so startlingly handsome, so poised and well-

continued

spoken. I'd never been more proud of you or myself for doing all that we were doing.

By then, you were also working at Project Inform *and* doing individual HIV counseling. And you were so good at *all* of it.

Then, of course, came the World AIDS Day Display in Oslo, Norway that December. What an incredible trip that was! One of those magic times in our lives when it all came together. You were so proud to be invited to the land of your ancestors as an AIDS expert. And remember all the fuss we caused at the hotel because we insisted on a double bed? The press conference was very successful. Again I was bursting with pride at the sight of you, looking more Norwegian than most of the Norwegians, smiling that gorgeous smile, flashing those baby blues, and looking like the picture of health, flooring all those reporters and government officials as you spoke openly and candidly as a person with AIDS.

In those days, it really seemed that we could change things. And that, somehow, we would be protected—we were working much too hard on things far too important to have time to falter. We thought that if we all just sewed fast enough, we could stop the epidemic. People would finally understand. Our government would finally care and act. We could save our friends. We could save you.

In the end, of course, we could not. The unthinkable happened—and now you, too, have fallen I love you, Garth Wall. You are the love of my life. You *are*, even now. I cannot put that love into the past tense. And you know, I'm so sick of hearing people talk about AIDS as a gift. It's not a gift, it's a damn nightmare. *You* were the gift—a gift I'll treasure and hold in my heart and soul forever. And I will make a panel for you, I promise. But not yet. I just can't let go yet.

With all my love,

Scoobie
(Danny Sauro)

I would like to tell you about Wade Welch, my third son. Wade brought some magic and laughter into our home. He went through our small Arizona town school system in the same grade as our son, Skip. The boys became good friends and when Wade's parents moved to California because of job opportunities, Wade moved in with us for his senior year of high school. This time was the beginning of Wade's career as a clown. He performed at schools, birthday parties, civic organizations, etc. He also became an integral part of our busy, active farm family.

After high school, Skip went to the University of Arizona and Wade continued to pursue his career by moving to Los Angeles and attending the Pasadena Play House School. He continued to "clown" while dreaming of a breakthrough in show business. When both boys arrived in our small town for their tenth high school reunion, I noticed that Wade looked pale and thin and when I received a call from Skip telling us that Wade had AIDS, I was devastated. Wade lived for two years bravely fighting the Kaposi's Sarcoma that was distorting his body and making his breathing very difficult.

I visited Wade as often as was possible and we spent many hours laughing and talking about his growing-up years in Coolidge. We not only talked about his life but about his death, and his dealing with loss . . . As I sat with Wade for the last time, I remember how important it was to me that he not feel on the outside, grotesque and unloved. I still saw the handsome young man with the beautiful brown eyes as I hugged him to me. It was and is VITAL that we help the suffering to know the human dignity that transcends any physical deterioration.

. . . In the long goodbye that is AIDS, I will never forget my short-term son, Wade.

Beth Cole

October 15, 1990

Dan was the son of my mother's cousin, Mildred. I did not know him well, but I remember him clearly. He may have been the first gay person I ever met, although I did not know he was gay at the time I met him. I was in junior high when he moved to Chicago to teach art history at the University of Illinois, Chicago Circle campus. My parents befriended him, which meant he came over for dinner occasionally, and that they let him store some of his things at the house when he moved out of town (fancy art magazines, a pedestal from a Greek column, etc.). He was neat and trim and cultured. He was from "back East," which was automatically alluring. Then, he had a kind of mystery about him, something I couldn't place, that both intrigued and scared me. He was unmarried, which surprised me. I didn't have a word for being gay at the time, yet at some level, I think I understood.

Dan only lived in the Chicago area for a short time, and he passed out of my immediate thoughts. It wasn't until a few years ago, when my parents received a letter from him, that he was jolted back into my consciousness. He wrote my parents, thanking them for their kindness years ago. He mentioned that a very close friend of his had recently died from a mysterious form of cancer for which there was no cure, and we all knew immediately that he was talking about AIDS.

I had come out as a lesbian years ago, and wanted to contact him, but I put it off. He was living in the New York area, not so far from me, yet I couldn't come up with the words to explain who I was. "Guess what? I'm a lesbian!" I was afraid he'd say "So what?" or "Just because I have AIDS, it doesn't mean I'm gay." I feared that we wouldn't have anything in common, that I would somehow offend him by taking this liberty. So I never got around to writing, and eventually my family read in his obituary that he was found dead in his apartment.

Dan was estranged from his mother. I never knew why, but I certainly suspect it was because she wouldn't accept his homosexuality. I remember hearing him say "The word 'mother' is not in my vocabulary." It was a chilling remark for a preteen to hear, and it chills me, even now, to think of it. It was so definite, and so final. How I wish I had contacted him, and that I could have asked him to explain.

I am afraid to contact his mother . . . fearing that perhaps the word "son" is absent from her vocabulary as well. I can say that he was raised in Philadelphia, that I believe he went to Harvard, that he had an M.A. in art history and architectural history, that he was a professor and curator, that he taught at the University of Illinois and Notre Dame, that he lived in those

continued

places, and in Jersey City. He was a curator at a museum in Reading, Pennsylvania. He was accused of stealing and was fired from his job. Later, he successfully sued them and received some settlement. I think he was living in Riverdale, New York, when he died.

Apparently his lover had already passed away when Dan became ill. Some family member told me that he had had an AIDS buddy, but he sent them away. He died alone. I think about the anger and bitterness he seems to have had, and I wonder how he would have responded if I had contacted him. I'll never know.

I tell this story and I sewed the panel to honor Dan's memory, and to hope that he can, in some way, know and be comforted that he is remembered.

Myrna Greenfield

This quilt is made in memory of my brother Doug, who died in Miami in 1986 . . .

Doug never really accepted himself and therefore refused to believe that we, his family, did. He didn't tell us he had AIDS—his lover called when it was evident Doug was dying. We all went to be with him. I feel that in those last days, he believed us. He was our Doug, a kind, gentle, beautiful man who did not deserve the hell he put himself through.

We love you, Doug, and miss you. The whole family has put that love into this quilt, even those you never knew or were too young to remember you.

The tears are always close to the surface, the pain so sharp, the lonesomeness a never-ending ache. The only comfort is that you don't hurt anymore . . .

Please list the quilt as Sweet Charity—D.B. Hopefully his friends will recognize it as his.

Thank you,

Diane R. Foster

August 11, 1989

Sgt. Rick Fenstermaker, USMC ══════

I first met Rick on March 20, 1987 in Portsmouth, Virginia. In a very short period of time, Sgt. Rick Fenstermaker, USMC, became my best friend and my family. I very strongly believe that if it weren't for Rick I would have taken my own life. My first HIV test results were returned positive—false positive. I saw no further need to live after that. Rick became my reason. This complete stranger gave my life new meaning. New hope. Out of the two-and-a-half years we knew each other I only have one letter from him. I always knew that he was thinking about me. Whenever something was going bad for me, he'd call. If it was going OK, he'd say, "I knew you were going to call me today." Rick is the type of person that every gay man looks to take home to Mother. I never could get him home to meet mine, but they knew each other's voices on the phone. My mom helped me create my best friend's panel.

I can only think of one way to describe how I felt, and still feel, about Rick:
"If anyone should ask me
to give a reason
why I loved my friend,
there could only be one answer:
    'Because he was he,
    because I was I.'"
                                    —*Montaigne*

Looking back on all the people that I have dated, Rick is the only person that I can say with all truth and honesty that I have fallen in love with. We never dated. Since his death on Dec. 1, 1989, any time that something has gone wrong in my life I have felt this "presence" around me and knew it was Rick trying to guide me into the right path. Even if you had just met Rick, he'd give you the shirt off his back.

The best way to describe him is with the two poems on his panel. The pink one is from Sonnet 116, by William Shakespeare. The second is from me.

Rick is the first person that I knew who died from AIDS. Since then I lost one other friend. I miss Rick. If I could have given him one more breath on this earth, I would have given him my life.

Mark A. Hannay

Van was my son's companion for about eight years.
They had an endearing relationship. When my son
became ill and was diagnosed with AIDS, Van was
there for him, with him, supporting and consoling him
and caring for him through the 21 months until his
death. Then, having also been diagnosed, Van
persevered through his own difficult times, supported
by the caring community of friends who had also been
a major part of my son's caregiving support system.

Van was a gentle and quiet person, although gifted
with a great sense of humor. He spent most of his
time away from his stressful job on a stock exchange
creating and nurturing a beautiful array of flower beds:
They were all around their house, in hanging planters
on the porch, in pots on the steps and floor areas of
the porch. The beauty of the flowers, and the serenity
of the garden area, were a great source of pleasure
and comfort to Van, and to all of his friends.

I came to know Van after my son's diagnosis,
through many telephone conversations (there was a
distance of 3,000 miles between our homes). I came
to care for him for the special person he was. I
transferred my limited opportunities for caring support
from my son at his death to Van and to his needs,
throughout his 20 months of illness after my son died,
until his own death.

During my son's illness, he told me about the Quilt, and asked that I look over the material and consider whether it might be something that I might want to do. I did, without hesitation, assure him that I knew I would want to make a panel for him. When the time came and I did make his panel, it proved to be, as I am sure is the case for everyone who creates a panel for a loved one, or even for a person not known to the maker, an intense grieving process, a vital step in getting through the heartache and grief of losing my son. When I began to work on Van's panel, it was, again, a source of "letting go" while wanting so badly to hang on.

I present this panel for Van with love and appreciation for all he was, and for all he did for my son.

My son was Dan McKenney. It is my hope that it will be possible for his panel to be placed together with Van's in a section of the Quilt, for any future displays at Seattle, Washington, which was their home community for the eight years they were together.

Eileen S. McKenney

ROBERT PATRICK LEWIS ════════

I first met Bob in the summer of 1985. He was "break-dancing" as part of a youth theatre workshop. Physically he was very good and he had an incredible sense of rhythm. His mother, Gloria, stood on the sidelines and watched her son. Soon afterwards, Gloria came and spoke to me about Bob's illness . . . she told me he was a hemophiliac. He was very prone to bleeds in his joints. I couldn't believe he danced so well. Gloria was a very cautious mother with Bob, but she knew he had to make his own choices; he had to decide the limitations of his body . . .

Bob was a very talented artist, winning many awards in local art shows. He was very gifted on stage, performing in many of our community theatre productions. Bob's cartoon strip ran in the local newspaper. He also created a poster that won a contest in San Antonio and was distributed throughout the city. It read "You Can't Get AIDS By Being Someone's Friend." When Bob drew the poster, he knew his own fate, but he didn't sign his work because of fear.

I created the panel using some of Bob's artwork. His last drawing is so poignant . . . I wanted to share it with as many people as possible . . .

The descriptive words on the panel are how I want Bob remembered . . . When I said he was a student, Gloria said we must include "teacher," because we learned so much about life from him. I am honored to have been his friend.

David L. Cockerell

My name is Mitzi Fleischer and I am Mikel Blue's aunt . . . Over the past three years, the dreadful AIDS disease brought Mikel and me very close. At last we were able to discuss it more openly. I visited him in July 1989 in Los Angeles, went with him to the support group Center of Living, shared a lot of his pain and disillusion. We both knew we wouldn't see each other again. He gave me a lovely memento that was given to him from another AIDS friend who since passed on . . .

One thing he was annoyed with me [about]: When I tried to assure him of a possible cure or a miracle drug that might help. But he knew better and wanted to talk about facts. His cousin suggested to me to ask his opinion of the Quilt. He seemed surprised at my question, but delighted—relieved. His response: "Would you really do this for me?" When I assured him, he said, "Please be sure there'll be a zebra on it!"

So the project of the quilt materialized. The artist in our family started with the zebras, sent it on to me, and all the busy hands started to act. I lovingly put it all together, every stitch with a heavy heart full of memories. As sad as the occasion it is made for, it is most gratifying to know that all his loving friends and family had the opportunity to express their feelings . . . so it will remain a living memorial to Mikel among our family and friends.

Kindest regards,
Mitzi Fleischer

January 23, 1990

JENNY B.

I first met this wonderful woman (who was to become my best friend) shortly after returning to college and although there was a difference in our ages it was never of any importance to either of us (I am 20 years older). Jenny conducted a workshop for paraprofessional counselors that I attended. And her warm friendly personality drew my interest and desire to know her. And I had that very good fortune from 1979 to 1985.

There are so many wonderful memories of this SPECIAL LADY that I would love to share, but neither time nor space will permit, but I would like to share these as they tell so much about her. We had talked and planned and looked forward to seeing "Cats" at the Shubert Theatre in Century City in July 1985, and although I knew she was ill, I was not prepared for how thin and frail she had become in a few weeks.

Anyway, we got to the theatre and Jenny and my

daughter and I really loved the show that we had been looking forward to for nine months. But as great as it was, the memory that made my heart sing was watching Jenny dance on the stage during intermission when the public was invited to meet the actors. When Jenny returned to her seat glowing with happiness, she said, "At last, my dreaming of dancing at the Shubert came true."

She entered St. Vincent Hospital two days later and remained in I.C.U. for three months before the end. But even with that she continued to give to me and my family. She arranged to have her Christmas gifts given to us and other friends before Christmas, because as she said, "It is a day in the heart—not the calendar."

Sleep well, sweet friend, you are missed.

Karen Barbara Dalyea

Dear Brothers and Sisters in the
NAMES Project,

It is very hard to describe the life of a good friend within a very few lines. It is harder to describe the feeling of loss at his passing. I believe that these will be more eloquently represented in the panel I made then I could ever cover in words.

When he died last year, I never grieved. I tried for a long time to forget—because it was too painful to remember. But when I saw your logo ''Remember My Name,'' I realized that I must remember—for his sake.

Land never told his parents that he was gay, or that he had AIDS. They still do not know. So I did not include his last name, in respect for his wishes.

Land was a great friend. The best. His concern for others, when he had little himself, his sympathy for others and their suffering, in the face of his own suffering, epitomizes his personality and his character.

He was gentle and kind. He was a black man who knew no color. He was Land . . .

When Land entered the hospital for what he thought was a routine checkup, we spoke on the phone almost every day. Within a week, he was in intensive care. I was barred from seeing him. Three months later, he was dead. I promised I would visit him, but could not. His death came as a shock I could not deal with, so I never went to his funeral.

My panel, I hope, will be the goodbye I never had time to say. A woman friend, whose son I taught a number of years ago, sewed this panel together. She spent many hours working on a memorial to a man she never met. I thank her for that.

The silhouette on this panel is almost an exact likeness of him. It has allowed me to see him at last— and to mourn. I love him. I'll miss him.

Chris B.

July 19, 1989

Dear Al,

I went to see the NAMES Project AIDS Memorial Quilt display at Rutgers today and missed you all over again. It was a very moving and impressive display but sad because it represents so many young lives that have been snuffed out. With renewed feelings, I once more was reminded, painfully, that never again will I see your face, kiss you, hear you speak my name, and just talk with you.

I've tried not to recall memories because it makes me sad and remorseful for precious time I didn't spend with you when I might have, for things I could have said and didn't and just to let you know I really did care, though I didn't always say so. My memories of us as brother and sister were a love/hate relationship, which I think is average. Sometimes I didn't understand why you did the things you did and wished you hadn't. Other times I admired your caring and protectiveness of our family, your friends and helpless creatures. You never had any good breaks in life and you suffered so much both physically and mentally. I don't know why and I guess I won't till I die.

We had lots of good times Al, and the best, most lasting memories are of our trip to Italy. What a wonderful experience! Because of all the wonderful pictures you took, I can reminisce and be thankful we all went and shared so many special memories together.

Al, I love you, I miss you and I pray you're free from all the suffering on earth. Do you see Dad?

Please pray for me and Mom that we may keep your memory alive and fulfill our purpose on earth. I'm waiting for the day we'll all be together again.

All my love,

Rosemarie Bonomo

April 22, 1990

What can I say about Jay?

He was vibrant, flashy, grand and glamorous. He had longterm relationships with men and women and was dedicated to whoever he was with at the time. Jay was a dancer, not just the metaphor in life, but for a living—boy, could he hustle! Everyone waited and wanted to dance with Jay—he made us all feel like Ginger Rogers!

I remember one Christmas party when Jay showed up all in black with gold ribbons all over—he looked like an exquisite Christmas gift, the truth is, NO ONE looked, moved or interacted with the world like Jay!

After he got sick, very sick, he only worried about Christine, the woman he lived with. A lot of us spent long hours caring for Jay; he got sick very fast. He had an aunt named Thelma, in those long blurred hours near death when he slept, it seemed forever, Thelma and all of us played gin—she took every nickel we had—I think Jay would have thought that was funny— Thelma did.

Jay was lucky—when he moved from the world to whatever awaits him, he had his whole family in the room, as his father read the 23rd Psalm.

I send you this Quilt in his memory—the purple is for awareness, the splattered paint for his need to always add a touch of color—the mylar heart for our love of him, the black sequins for his glamour.

Add him to the thousands you have, for he would enjoy their company. We all miss him terribly.

Love to you, Jay!

Your friend,
Zak Haley

June 19, 1988

I have held this panel for 10 months. It seemed as though as long as I had it, it would bring my son home, but that is not to be, so I'm sending it to you in the hopes you will be able to display it in December with the rest of his friends.

Thank you,

Bette Smith
(mother)

Today is Frank's 36th birthday. Instead of making him a cake, though, I've been making him a panel, because, on the 3rd of June ("another sleepy dusty Delta day," as they say in "Ode to Billie Joe") Frank died of AIDS.

Frank Blanco was my best friend—we met on my very first day of high school, twenty years ago next month . . . There is no way I could ever put down on paper all the things I know about Frank and all that he meant to me.

His death has been and will be one of the great tragedies of my life, and for purely selfish reasons. I just wasn't ready to have him go away. I miss him. Someone tried to console me the other day, saying it would get easier—I hope it never does. I hope and pray that it will always hurt this much, and anger me this much, and that every AIDS death that follows is just as painful to me. I never want to get used to something this horrible.

Frank was a refugee from Cuba, coming here when he was 9 years old. Thank goodness, when he was 15, his family decided to move out of Washington, D.C., to suburban Arlington, to a house several blocks from mine. As I said, we met my first day of high school and were best friends ever since. We went our separate ways for a while—Frank was drafted and spent the Vietnam War typing for a chaplain in Fort Jackson, South Carolina.

In the late 1970s, I got a call here in San Francisco. Frank had just decided to move out here, and the proximity made our friendship stronger and more intense. After two years, he moved back to

Washington, to take care of his parents as they got older.

He was diagnosed with AIDS in 1984. In February of 1987, he collapsed from pneumocystis, and when his brother explained to the family what was wrong with him, the family responded with, "Of course we will take care of you." For the last year and a half of his life, Frank was taken care of by his 80-year-old parents and two aunts who lived with them. None of them had any medical training; only one of them spoke English. And they were absolutely amazing, learning how to do as much as possible so that Pancho (their nickname for him) would have to spend as little time as possible in the hospital. They think that everyone takes care of their sick children, and it is hard for me to make them realize what an incredible labor of love they performed, and how much Frank appreciated it.

Frank came down to the NAMES Project Quilt when it was in Washington in October of 1987. I had been working with the readers all day, and was being a brave little soldier—stiff upper lip and that sort of thing—as I was escorting readers to and from the stage as they read the names of the memorialized dead, so I felt I had to be as stoic as possible. But suddenly, there was Frank, and I knew that one day I would be making this quilt panel for him. I always told him that we didn't have enough time left together for me to waste it crying around him, but that day we cried and cried together. I told him I would make a panel for him, and he was glad about that. I said I wanted his other friends to help, rather than make it

continued

myself, and he liked that idea. I designed this quilt panel, drew it on a piece of cardboard, cut the cardboard apart, and sent templates to 16 of Frank's friends.

Frank was constantly surrounded by music. And of course, his favorite singers were the Supremes. At Frank's memorial service, which was shortened from the one that he had planned, for the sake of his parents, there was no music whatsoever. This seemed wrong to most of us, so I wanted to make sure that he has some memorial where the Supremes were always singing. That is why I have sewn a Walkman into my Quilt panel. On my section, there is a book of messages from various participants in this panel, and the quotes that Frank had picked out to be read at his memorial service. When this book is opened, it triggers a switch, and the Walkman plays "I Hear A Symphony," Frank's favorite Supremes song. Whenever someone visits his panels, there will be music.

Frank loved to sing, and he couldn't sing on key to save his soul, but somewhere, I know that imperfect soul is singing with perfect pitch.

Paul Hill

August 15, 1988

P.S.: And now for the anger stage. This is a wonderful panel, and I am very proud of it, but I hate it. I hate it so very much, because, instead of having Frank to talk to and laugh with and hold on to, all I have is this damn piece of fabric. It isn't enough and it isn't fair, and there isn't anything I can do about it.

I had a personal intention in preparing this patch of love. I made it, in part, in remembrance of him, a lifelong friend who died, according to his obituary, of cancer. Whether or not it was AIDS-related, I don't know. Could never ask his family. All that I do know is that he loved me steadfastly and that I could not find the courage to love him back.

Because my friend did not come out publicly, at least to my knowledge, I do not feel I can go into details about our aborted relationship. But if my friend had lived, he would be in his late fifties as I am. I came out at the age of 58, about the time I retired from a civil service job which I held for 25 years. Over these years, I carried the thought in the back of my mind, that once we both retired and I had fulfilled my family responsibilities, that we could get together, two silver foxes, and build that relationship which I know now we both wanted, but which I was afraid to go for. Only my friend had died.

It doesn't matter how. He's gone and I am the lonelier for it. I do know that some time after hearing of my friend's death, these words came to me. Have not left me:

Love, freely offered, once refused, may never come again.

And I want to say, don't let this happen to you. Go for it.

Edward Zalewski

To the NAMES Project,

For some reason this letter about the enclosed panels is harder to do than the panels themselves. I imagine it is the final giving up of my memories to combine with memories of so many others.

I know that most panels have only one name, and I understand your request around this. So I will try and explain my multi-name panels.

I have been professionally and personally involved in the epidemic since 1981—I visited the Quilt this past winter in a fugue of desperate feelings— overwhelmed by death, systems that didn't work, never ending crisis and a terrible isolation. Along with all of this was an always present need to keep alive the memories and names of those I loved who died.

Being with the Quilt allowed me safety for my grief, hope in people's continued caring and the knowledge that I could put my names and memories someplace where they would be protected and known. I decided to do a panel for those I loved who died. In the months it took to formulate an idea I lost many more friends and now send you two panels.

Every time a death reaches into my life I feel as though another piece of my heart has been taken away—it made me always think of Janis Joplin singing "Heartbreaker" and suddenly I "had" the panels. Please hang them side by side as they are really one.

Thank you for providing this memorial, for allowing a place for us to sigh our private and collective grief—and for hope that there will be a day when the last panel is hung!

Susan Messinger Black

Thoughts about Benjamin:

He was born on April 19, 1979, beginning the world in typically dramatic fashion: 36 hours of labor, with his mother pledging "No more children!" At six months he was diagnosed with hemophilia, again dramatically, with a spinal bleed and paralysis. The doctors were unsure as to whether he would ever be able to walk—but walk, and run he did, with a fierce love of life and an infectious joy of living.

He made his way through preschool hemophilia, with mouth bleeds, knee bleeds, bleed bleeds. He learned to live with pain and tolerate it. It was a part of his world; he simply dealt with it and got on with the business of living.

The things he liked? Muffa, his teddy bear, who accompanied him constantly through life, and drawing. Legos, Saturday morning cartoons, stickers, and collecting—he had one of the few collections in Phoenix of fish eyeballs and teeth, compliments of his aunt in Norway! He loved school, and was fortunate in his final year at school to find a teacher who knew what he needed and didn't need. His favorite places were the island in Norway where he could catch crabs and *maybe* a lobster, the cabin in Pine, and San Diego—especially Sea World and Pacific Beach. His food tastes were eclectic: everything from Happy Meals to chicken livers on pasta with hollandaise sauce! And he *loved* his cats, Figaro and Barney.

The strongest thing he gave to all of us was his ability to rise above and confront his pain, his fear. By

continued

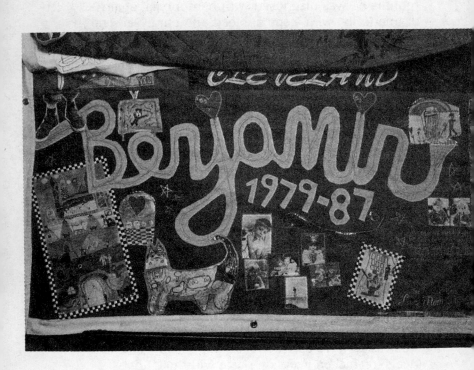

his example he enabled all of us who were a part of his life and death to accept our own pain and fear, and try to overcome it. That, along with the incorrigible joy with which he embraced life and living provided a model whose understanding showed the depths of which children are capable.

The drawing in the top right corner of the quilt is an illustration. He made this one while he was in the hospital, and he called it "The Magic Garden." He explained that you had to travel down this yellow brick road to get to it, and outside the gate was a nice man whose job it was to take care of all the beautiful flowers. In order to get inside you had to go through all these bars, and "it would be hard." But once you were through the bars, it was . . . rainbowland.

We love him and miss him . . . he is still very much with us.

Love,

Sonja and David Saar

Dear Tony:

Well, your panel for the Quilt is finished and it's my job to do the write-up. I thought that you would like to hear from all of us.

Marie, Kathy and Michael made the panel; and Michael and David videotaped it so that the Iron Cross members in Montreal could see it. Everyone here in Boston saw it while it was displayed at the 119. It goes without saying that it turned out great. The white leather letters, your club colors and those studs— WOW!

I did not want to write this alone so I did what we always did, planned a dinner date. Eddie, Marie, Kathy and I went to the European for pizza one night to talk about you. Don't worry, it was all good—what else could it be!

Eddie was saying how you would tell everyone that you were the oldest and wisest; but give us a break, it was only by three minutes! He said that the two of you were not only twins (triplets, if you count Betty) but more importantly you were best of friends.

When Eddie mentioned friends, that's when Kathy chimed in and started talking about how you would spontaneously call your friends up on the phone early in the morning and wake them up. Would you feel guilty? Never. You would just tell them, "Too bad, you sleep enough when you die." You don't know how much that attitude of yours has helped us. We know you're always here, just sleeping.

Then Marie started to talk (and talk, and talk) about your attitude toward the world and how much joy you got out of the simple things in life. She said that you had "the heart of a child and the soul of an angel." You were always the peacemaker and you would never want to hear people talk badly about others. Since you only saw the good in people, it was easy for us (and everyone) to be your friend.

With all of this talking going on (and me writing everything down), it gave me a chance to do some thinking. (I know—you told me I sometimes think too much. Don't worry, I'm getting better.) What I thought about was your attitude toward life. Kathy said it best, "He always made the best out of the cards he was dealt." You did; and when things start to make me crazy I just think, "How would Tony react to this?" Boy, that calms me right down and also puts a smile on my face.

Well, "Buddy," I have to honestly say that we miss you but we also know that you will always be with us. Thanks.

Oh, yes—what we also kept talking about was your great sense of humor. Thanks for all the laughs.

Take care and love,

Vincent G. Licenziato

I first met Kandi on Ward B-2 at Fairmont Hospital in 1986. That was the first time she had been there. I remember her telling me about a hospital where they put her food tray outside the door once because they were afraid of AIDS. That was previous to Fairmont Hospital.

I never knew her before she was sick but we talked about growing up a lot and we had a lot in common. I also saw her and her mother reunite during one of Kandi's many hospital stays. There were a lot of people in and out of the hospital who helped care for and grew to love Kandi.

Many times I heard from medical personnel that she was not going to recover from her current hospital stay. Then she would be up and walking in a couple of days and the doctors were baffled. She was very proud of her comebacks and used to say that God was keeping her alive for a reason. I think it was to help people because she helped me.

Her proudest moment was when she greeted Mother Teresa with flowers when Mother Teresa visited The Center in Oakland. It meant a lot to her.

Periodically when she got a pass to leave the

hospital or I picked her up from where she was staying at the time, we would go out to eat or go see a movie together. We would talk a lot and our talks helped me understand myself.

Sometimes she stayed with me. We were like a couple of little kids. Once we ate pizza and almost died laughing watching a Pee-Wee Herman movie. When she stayed with me or we went out, Kiska (my Siberian husky) would shadow her. Kiska never left Kandi's side and they slept together when Kandi visited me. They were inseparable. One time, I sneaked Kiska on into Kandi's room (don't tell anyone) on the ward and it was quite a reunion.

In the last couple of days of Kandi's life near the end of 1988 I talked to her a lot and didn't get much response. At that time, I told her I was going to sneak Kiska into the room and I got a big smile. That smile meant a lot to me and Kiska and I miss her.

Lyman Ditson

P.S.: Kiska moved, and one of her pawprints smudged but I think Kandi would have said that it was OK.

JOHN A. BORDA ═══════════════════

I loved Johnny Borda. Johnny was one of the nicest guys I ever met in my life. Had I been more mature at the time I lived with Johnny, he might not be where he is today.

He was kind, loving and brought much joy to my life. I can still picture you, Johnny, in the kitchen making homemade gravy with it splattering all over the walls, baking a gingerbread house at Christmastime with more flour on you and the floor than there was in the gingerbread house, and of course, the time I came home and you had two sheep dogs in the apartment in addition to Shag—all because the animal shelter said they would be put to sleep if no one adopted them.

Johnny, I've always felt whoever you were with never really appreciated your love. I know I didn't and I hope some day (in a better place) I can make it up to you.

Love you always,

T.E.M.

P.S.: The poem you gave me one week after we were together, I now give back with the same love with which it was given:

"Oh God please comfort and watch over me,
And help me solve this mystery,
I'm happy now but yet I'm sad,
I love, I lose, I hope and pray,
I've steered my life on different roads,
I stop, I go and stop and go,
I cry, I laugh then laugh again and cry,
I reach out and touch but afraid to hold,
I walk then I run, I can smile again,
but I fall, I wake once more,
Only to find it's still the same."

Robert Jules Muhlfelder was raised against his will in Holidaysburg and Harrisburg, Pennsylvania. Jules was Bob then, bright where it meant trouble, gay where it meant God knows what, an oddball beatnik theater person seemingly exiled to a world intent on living out the facade of Ozzie and Harriet placidity.

He did find a friend, a vivacious girl fighting her own battle, rebelling in her own way, and she became, as did everyone who entered Jules' world with any comprehension of him, a lifelong friend.

At the age of 14, Jules was shipped off to summer camp and discovered he was neither crazy nor alone. By a happy coincidence this camp had also attracted the loyalty of a group of proudly precocious New Yorkers, self-styled bohemian cosmopolites, cynical idealists, infatuated with protest marches, theater, and obscure R&B. And these kids liked him, understood and appreciated his gift for finding the short, simple, absurd but well-concealed hypocrisies that make life dull, the posturings that Jules found with the speed of a ferret. Jules knew that he had a voice that was his own, admired by the people he admired, and that he had a home in New York.

He settled there as soon as possible, first as a student at NYU, where he felt a little worse about dropping out than most, and then as an acting student, complete with portfolio and 8 × 10″ glossies, less an attempt at stardom than to remake himself.

Plunging into the '60s, and never a man to deny himself drugs, booze, irresponsible decisions, and sudden crazy plans, he did all of that. Excess was one

continued

of his lifelong, thoroughly unfulfilled impulses. It was a strange contrast with Jules' grave, pensive, deeply held belief in loyalty, careful listening, and the forms and obligations of politeness.

In those years, the years he also started having sex with men, Jules was lucky enough to have found a great love, an intensely passionate, intellectual, and highly accomplished actor named Jim, who died after a few years of cancer. Perhaps because of this man, Jules had a blessedly short struggle with himself over his sexuality, and enthusiastically welcomed the coming of gay pride and sexual liberation. Jules was a man who definitely believed in kissing on the first date.

With Jim's death, Jules felt that life had turned an abrupt corner. He became Jules instead of Bob, and decided that the self-promotion and obsession necessary to be an actor wasn't in him. He traded life in the theater for life in the kitchen, using charm in lieu of experience to obtain a position at the Waldorf-Astoria, where he soon rose to sous chef, and then went on to the Cornell Club.

In 1973, Jules moved to San Francisco, eventually becoming the co-owner of Reality Sandwiches. He in fact became sandwich-maker to the poets, of whom there were many in San Francisco at the time. Unfortunately, wonderful as the sandwiches were, they were priced low enough to finally drive the sandwich-makers out of business.

Jules reached the conclusion that if he desired to continue some level of spontaneity and excess in his personal life, he needed a commensurate amount of security and stability in his professional life, and so he joined the civil service. He landed a job with Social Security, where he worked diligently for the remainder of his life.

But after a while, the mellow tranquility of San Francisco life began to grate on Jules, and he found himself missing the sharper edge of the people and pace of New York. Unfortunately, his financial situation precluded a relocation. Toward the end of a hard week, his remaining discretionary income barely enough for a single drink, Jules set off for his favorite bar. He was slowly sipping his lone cocktail with the wan hope that a friendly compatriot might buy him another, when a large stereo speaker fell off the wall and hit him in the head. The insurance settlement from this completely unprovoked but fortuitous attack was sufficient to finance his return to New York.

In 1987 Jules found what he knew would be, could be, a gem of an apartment. His gem was one hundred square feet in size, plastered with pinups and rotting cork, and featured exposed pipes and strange gunk on the floor—but it was, as Jules pointed out, on a great block. And eventually, with care, and thought, and very little money, it did turn into a gem of an apartment on a very nice block.

In 1987, Jules also tested HIV positive. Almost until the end of his life, Jules worked and laughed and drank and belted out show tunes and went out and saw friends and went on living his life.

Friends of Jules Muhlfelder

CLARENCE ROBINSON, JR. ══════

I had returned home in late fall, having spent the summer months at my mountain home in North Carolina. The first evening that I had to visit my friends, they told me about a 23-year-old who was quite seriously ill with AIDS. He was in the county hospital, was not being given any treatment, was placed in an open hallway and everyone avoided him, except one gay nurse. I learned that the only family member who came to see him was his divorced father, who was extremely upset about the way the medical people were (not) treating his son.

Hearing about this young man certainly cut to my bones, as my one son is only one year older than Clarence. At that time I was attending my first meetings with a local group which was trying to support persons with AIDS. Clarence's father was asked to attend one of our meetings and it was truly a shock to see this burly, roughcut, unskilled phosphate mine worker as he talked (and cried) about the mistreatment of his son. This man had tried every possible way to get medical help for his son, but none was forthcoming.

Unfortunately, I never met Clarence Jr. He died before I could visit him. My friends who went to visit him quickly learned that one did not have a quick visit with him. He was terribly lonely and would use any ploy to stretch out the visit. His favorite trick was, as his visitors were leaving, to request that they drive to McDonald's and bring him a hamburger and a Coke. Then he'd want them to stay till he finished eating.

A Friend of PWAs

John Kennedy was a beloved and favorite teacher—a break in my monotonous junior high school day and a reason to look forward to Wednesday afternoons—that was the day designated for my singing lessons.

Those afternoons were, then, so taken for granted. I guess I assumed I would be the one to break them off when it came time to find another teacher or go to college, or whatever . . .

Once Mr. Kennedy became ill, he retired from his teaching job at school; most weeks, though he was still up to the Wednesday lessons. For some months, we were working on a song I was going to perform at a school concert—I'm not sure if he thought I sang it well or not. The evening of the concert came and he was in the audience watching me. I wanted so much to make him proud. "Okay," I thought as I sang, "here comes the last phrase; do it for him."

At intermission I saw my mentor. "Well?" I said. "Beautiful!" was the whisper from his mouth. I'll never forget that night.

I think of Mr. Kennedy often and of what he represents to me. He was a person who really made a difference—not only in my life, but to many students before my time. So few people can truly be said to have made things better . . . well, he did. He made them care.

Vicki Shabo

This is the hard part—put your son on paper—sum up 27 years in two pages.

Joe's sister, Molly, couldn't do it. They were so close and such good friends—but she just could not—it's too soon.

So I'll tell you that mostly Joe's friends remember his humor and his smile. Also they remember that there was never a dull moment with Joe around—I believe they call it a "mover and shaker." Their contributions for his banner recalled his love for New York (a seven-year resident before coming home to California)—his love of dry martinis and knowing it was 5 o'clock somewhere—his cat "B" and "B's" love of raw eggs—his love of travel—anywhere (it was his job, too). His family—well, we just loved him and always will.

His epitaph—Laughter shared is Love never lost—Loving still beyond Goodbye.

My contribution to his flag was an eye—closed—with a very large teardrop. We all miss the color that was Joe.

Shirley Reid

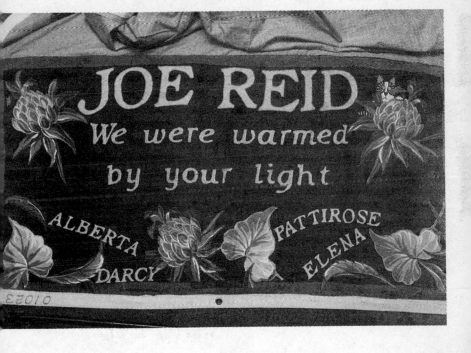

I only saw Larry once. I went to his apartment to visit and I noticed that the walls were filled with framed blueprints and architectural drawings. The clean lines of the drawings reminded me of his sensitive, articulate personality.

We spoke on the phone after that and started to become close when he was taken into the hospital. He died very suddenly and unexpectedly.

James Latus

DAVID LEE MANDELL, JR.

David was born eight weeks premature in Dundee, Scotland, and from the beginning of his life, he showed everyone who knew him what it was to live.

Diagnosed at nine months with classic severe hemophilia, he was still able to enjoy the most that life could offer. As he grew and developed both physically and emotionally, his family was aware of a specialness about him.

Colors, sounds and odors were intense and to be enjoyed to the maximum possible. The child was unable to walk. Even with the pain of joint bleeds sometimes in both ankles, his gait was always "full speed ahead." Crutches and a wheelchair did nothing to slow him down.

His interests ran a gamut of all that fell in his path. Computer, space, coins, music, arcade games, and even participating in the cooking of his mother. He loved bikes, skates, cartoons, bathroom humor, chess, the San Diego Symphony and riding in the rain.

His favorite foods were spaghetti, steak, strawberries, melon, all types of seafood (especially lobster and Alaskan king crab) and chocolate (until the end when his system could not tolerate the richness of it).

He had no concern for fads in fashion but loved a special jacket which was seldom removed. ALF was a special favorite of his and he felt a kinship with the alien character because, I guess, like David, he was different.

continued

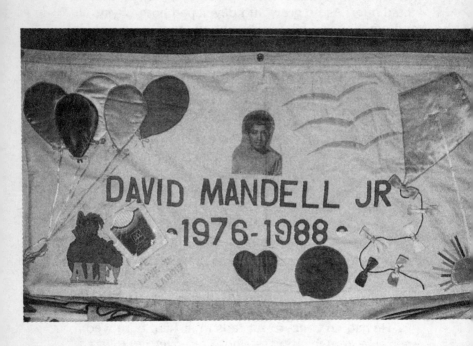

DAVID LEE MANDELL, JR.

He felt something special for a particular girl in his class but went with her name unrevealed. It was one of the very few things that he held secret.

He hated being a hemophiliac but in spite of that, did better than most in coping with it. He hated having AIDS but, even knowing he was to die, was more concerned for the comfort and ease of his family and friends.

David was my son, but he did not belong to me. He was himself always and what a special thing that was. I cannot think of David without aching for that specialness. He made all who knew him better than they thought they could be.

Suzi Mandell

May 6, 1988

Gary Mannor lived in the Egypt of the Pharaohs. He was of noble birth and rested until his next life in a pyramid. His next life was that of a mother in a primitive pacific culture. In that life he was disfigured in some way and became an outcast.

This life was no kinder to Gary. A lively, boisterous, colorful man, he became an interior designer. Gary drew on those previous lives in his profession, preferring elegant displays juxtaposed with primitive artifacts. Everything he touched became more beautiful. He was so talented. He could do anything with his hands . . . needlepoint to woodcarving, upholstery to landscaping—his life was devoted to making the world more beautiful. And despite becoming disfigured and outcast again in this life, Gary left this world more beautiful through his very presence.

And Gary, when you tell stories about me wherever you are, make them laugh as much as I did!

David Cullen Powers

This panel is dedicated to my husband, Kirk. I was lucky, indeed, to have had Kirk's love in my life for 13 wonderful years—the last eight of which I was honored to be his wife. We were just starting our lives together when Kirk had an accident and had to have several blood transfusions. We had no idea then that the blood supply was unsafe or that he was at risk.

Kirk was diagnosed in January 1989, and lived almost two years. He loved life to the fullest and realized how precious life was. . . .

I wanted very much to create a panel in his honor which would reflect Kirk—so that the people who knew him could smile and remember and those who didn't know him could get a glimpse of who he really was. So I set his panel in a place he loved, the park, and incorporated some of the things he loved most in this life. Kirk loved riding his Harley. In fact, his last wish was to get to ride a Harley one more time. Some very special Harley riders and Kirk's buddy made this last Harley ride a reality for him.

Kirk had three chow dogs which all played an important part in his life. I know he would have wanted Sport, Scout, and Slick to be with him forever in the park with his Harley . . .

To commemorate Kirk's whimsical spirit, I have a teddy bear picnic with his three favorite teddy bears. Kirk loved to play bass guitar, so the guitar is leaning against the tree as if Kirk just left it there. Lastly, the heart on the tree symbolizes the eternal love Kirk and I shared which I will carry in my heart forever.

Linda S.

ANDREW

Writing about making the panel for Andrew is
almost as difficult as it was to make it—and made
more complicated by the fact that we made several
panels for Andrew for me to take to the Quilt Project
in Thailand, in the U.K., France, Holland, New
Zealand, and, of course, the NAMES Project in the U.S.
Andrew was the founder, together with Richard
Johnson, of the Australian Quilt Project. As much as
one can be, I, as a friend, was prepared for Andrew's
death. We had seen him become gradually weaker
and weaker over a number of months. What I was not
prepared for was the effect on me of losing him as the
founder of the Quilt Project. I felt an enormous sense
of responsibility and loneliness—even with a
wonderful and supportive Quilt committee.

Andrew was, in many respects, a difficult person
to love in the sense that he found it very difficult to
express personal feelings and emotions. I felt very
valued and loved by Andrew, but it was rarely spoken.
I relied on him heavily when he became too ill to
continue with the running of the Quilt. A few months
before he died, Andrew decided to move back to live
with his sister and her family in Perth. During the
week that I was in Perth, Drew became more and
more frail and eventually his legs would not move.
The day I left Perth to return with the Quilt to Sydney,
I went to say goodbye to Andrew. As we hugged each
other, Drew said to me, "Well, see you next time the

Quilt's in Perth." Andrew died about two weeks later. It took me a long time to accept the anger and disappointment I felt at that farewell.

When we started making the panels for Andrew, we would work very well on the background of the quilt—until it came to writing his name—and I found I could not do it. I would wait until another member of the Quilt Committee sewed or painted his name. The panel that we made for the NAMES Project Quilt is modeled on the one that Andrew and a group of his friends made for the Project a few years ago—"For all our Aussie mates." Andrew's panel is green and gold—the Australian colors, and his name is made with teddy bear material as a tribute to his collection of over 100 teddy bears. . . .

As time goes on I could write endlessly about Andrew, his little giggle, his sense of fun, and his passion for the Quilt Project. Now I am afraid I would start crying and not be able to stop . . . and there is so much work to be done . . .

With love,

Libby Woodhams,
Former convenor,
Australian AIDS
Memorial Quilt Project

Craigton A. Kim was known to the world as "Craig" and known to me as "Puppy." Our pet names. He was the "Puppy," and I was "Thumper," and who can tell how nicknames just kind of stick when you least expect them to.

Born of Chinese and Korean parentage, Craig was an amazing blend of cultures. Although totally American in his demeanor, he loved and never forgot the history behind his being. Fortunately for me, he was quick to share the wonderful mysteries of that history.

Quick of gleeful wit, he giggled when I first struggled to learn the art of handling kim chee with chopsticks. But he insisted that I continue my learning process and introduced me to a whole world that I had hardly dared to hope to know. My introduction to his Asian culture included an exposure to a remarkable and amazing lesson in respect. That included his respect for his family, for whom he cared greatly, for his heritage, which he never let slip from his grasp, and a respect for his friends, who will remember him always for the many ways in which he touched their lives. I can only pray to be able to pass on the lesson of respect that he gave to me so that it can touch the lives of others as it touched mine.

It is out of my respect for Craig's memory and a sincere respect for his wonderful family that I offer this quilt. It has been prepared in a manner in which I feel he would have approved. Inspired by the little red Chinese envelope known as a Lychee, which is given out at Chinese New Year as a token of good fortune for the year to come, the quilt is an impression of what Craig would have wanted to give to the world: Red for the good luck he would have wanted us to have. Gold for the worldly fortunes to which he knew we all aspire. The wisdom of the monkey for the Chinese year of his birth. A few words in memory of the "little things" that he loved so much.

As I have said on the quilt itself, Thumper misses the Puppy. But he has left behind gifts of knowledge that will never be forgotten.

Barry A. Cardoza,
a.k.a. "Thumper"

August 15, 1988

Dear David,

I was thinking about you today and thought I'd write. One of the things that I was thinking about is how much the mothers of your childhood friends loved your gentleness and kindness, even as a small boy. Oh! how they loved your giggle! I'm so glad that little giggle turned into an infectious laugh as you grew into a caring young man.

Do you remember Piddles and Wiggles? It seems I can hardly look at animals without being reminded of how much you enjoyed the rabbits, pigeons, guppies, hamsters, cats, dogs, and especially how you loved those twin goats! Did you finish the aquarium yet? I know you were working hard on it one of the last times we talked. . . .

Are you and Rich working on a set right now? I remember how great your sets looked in "Angel Dusted." Gave me a chance to brag to all my friends. I am proud of you, you know.

I'm so glad that you and Connie took that trip to Seattle a few years ago . . . just for fun! Just to think a brother and sister really got along so well (even though I remember all those arguments when you were kids), that you would actually want to take a vacation together! That's great. And Amber is so enjoying all the shells you brought back for her. . . .

At the reception following your service we had the best time eating good food and remembering you and looking at the bright neon cactus you made for your dad. It was a really special time. The balloons were great, too, floating off after the service. You'd have really enjoyed it.

Love,
*Wanda Peabody
(Mom)*

Michael was a wonderful son and brother. . .

Michael was a very hard worker and wanted very much to go to college and become a lawyer. When he found out he had AIDS, it was like everything changed for him. He worried he would hurt his family if anyone knew. He was afraid his family and friends would turn away from him and not want to be around him. No one should live that way—afraid of losing their job, family and friends. . . .

God bless all of the wonderful friends that stood by him until the end.

Marlene Sargent
(mother)

Lynn was a real sweet girl who got AIDS very early in life, at 18 years old. Lynn was a street person when we met her, and she brought joy and sorrow into our lives. Lynn loved life, she loved ducks, rabbits, and singing gospel and country music.

Lynn had a very hard life but she fought her way through till the very end.

Lynn has a little four-year-old son who has AIDS that she gave up at the age of two months because she knew she wouldn't be able to give him the care he needed. This took a lot of guts and love, to give up your own child, so he could have at least a chance!

Lynn's little boy is named Robbie and he is being adopted now by a very loving couple in North Carolina who love him a lot. Lynn is sadly missed by Gary Sheffield, Tom Rapp, her parents, Mr. and Mrs. Roger Silky, and little Robbie. But she lives on in all our hearts.

Gary Sheffield and
Tom Rapp

One of us knew Bobby for five years as best friend, project partner, fun conspirator, and "husband." The other of us knew him only for eight short months as ice cream maker, gentle man, and teacher.

Bobby was known by many as a strong, compassionate, and gentle teacher in this time of crisis. He was known for his articulate and moving visualization speeches, for his incredible media presence, for his empowerment of people with AIDS, for his refusal to be identified as a victim, for his openness and willingness to help others coping with diagnosis, and for his need to live rather than die with AIDS.

To us, Bobby was our pal. The little boy came out at strange hours . . . a call at midnight to ask if he was disturbing us . . . an insistence on having cookies in the house always and at all costs! . . .

Bobby's favorite saying was "Look for me in the rainbows!" His favorite song: "Somewhere Over The Rainbow." His favorite items: rainbow streamers, rainbow stained glass, rainbow flags . . . well, just about anything with a rainbow!

And so, we look for our friend in the rainbows!

Holly Smith and
Mary Russi,
panelmakers

This panel is for my friend, John Beard, who died in June 1987. He was a wonderful friend who loved unconditionally and always understood. He was a man who loved life and particularly enjoyed creating with his hands. A seeker of spiritual light, he reassured me, shortly before his death, that he would be there to greet me when I died. He was part of my life for a short time and yet had a great influence. We met at a Shanti support group. My brother was ill, and he had lost 13 friends. Gradually we became friends and I enjoyed the times we shared talking, laughing and crying about life.

He loved small animals and was especially attached to "Doggie," his pet of 15 years, who died in his arms. "Obi-Wan" was his chihuahua who came to live with him after "Doggie's" death and kept him company the last year of his life.

He always said "I love you" at the end of a telephone conversation, and I knew he meant it. He became my friend during an especially difficult time and because of his love I learned to love him and others affected by the epidemic.

I miss him more than I can express, but know he is and will always be in my heart.

Jacque Campbell

This panel has been prepared for our father, Richard Gordon Simmons. The NAMES Project has given us the chance to express feelings, emotions, and experiences which most people do not have the opportunity to share with others, especially after a loved one has physically left us. It offers a healing process no one can understand unless they too have been touched by its tragic cause and results.

Gordon Simmons lived in a northern California community at the time of his illness. He was very happily married to his wife and best friend of over 18 years. They were married on a beach near San Francisco in the early '70s (the era of love, peace, and magic). They had their little poodle named Groovy with them when they said their vows. Their love for this breed led them on a long journey, raising, showing, and breeding Gorgis standard poodles (Gorgis is their kennel name). They walked away with many champions through the years. They had a motor home which they drove to shows farther than their immediate area. Dad loved that motor home! His favorite dog, however, turned out to be a thoroughbred Chihuahua named Pistol. This dog won many honors and fell in lust with one of their standard poodles named Prissy. What a pair! And if owners are indeed like their dogs (or vice-versa) then I believe these animals were perfect for Dad! All of them had outgoing personalities, yet demanded their space.

It has taken one and a half years to get up the guts and perseverance to finish this panel. It's been worth all of the gathering, costs, and time to release our love for all to share. Please enjoy the bits and pieces of our father's life contained within this panel. It is only a tiny part of his existence, a glimpse and reflection of his life.

*Sharon J. Simmons and
April J. Simmons*

KURT ALAN KITCHEN ═══════════════

My name is Kurt Alan Kitchen, and I was born on March 2, 1959, in Calhoun County, Battle Creek, Michigan. I was the oldest of five children raised by my parents, Joseph and Gretta Kitchen.

In 1973, we moved to Houghton Lake, Michigan. There I attended Houghton Lake High School, eventually graduating with honors in 1977. During my years in high school I was involved in many projects and committees. It was easy for me to like everyone, and all my classmates seemed to like me. I was on the Homecoming Committee for three years and editor of the yearbook during my senior year. I was also involved with the drama class and was lead actor in a number of school plays. My fellow classmates during my senior year voted me as: "Most Likely to Succeed," "Best-Looking Guy," and "Best Personality." As busy and as active as I was in school and all the school activities, I chose to hold a job after school throughout my high school years. This allowed me to have the cars and boats that I loved very much and that all my friends enjoyed with me. I had a tremendous number of friends in Houghton Lake and those friends gave me a great deal of satisfaction throughout my short life.

1985 was a good year for me. I met and fell in love with a very special man named Keith. Keith lived in Flushing, Michigan, and by choice in 1986, I moved to Flushing to live with him. I was offered employment with a local florist. Finally, everything was going well with me. I was enjoying a lot of peace and happiness in my life.

In 1987, Keith was promoted and transferred to Boston.

Everything was wonderful, until October 1988, when I was diagnosed with PCP. I had AIDS! Now my world started crumbling around me. My employer terminated my employment, but continued to provide my health care benefits. Boredom was a major concern. Keith and I purchased a home in Boston which needed a great deal of tender loving care. Perfect for me. I became very busy remodeling and reconstructing parts of the house, with only a few guidelines to help me, which were obtained by working with my father on a few projects earlier in my life. Sewing came easy for me. I made all the draperies, bedspreads, and comforters. During all this time, I felt my body changing. I had good days and bad days, all the while becoming weaker. It was like going from a strong 30-year-old to a little old man within a year. My spirits were being constantly uplifted by all the compliments given to me by friends and relatives about the house and what I was able to do with it.

My last two months required 24-hour care. Mom knew that I needed her, so, with her and Keith's help, and a Boston Hospice, I was able to receive all my care at home, in the house that had given me so much pleasure.

I died on Tuesday, November 13, 1990, at Brigham and Women's Hospital with Mother at my side. By my request my body was cremated and my remains lie at rest in Memorial Park Cemetery, Battle Creek, Michigan.

Keith has since left Boston, returning to Houghton Lake, Michigan, where he currently resides, along with my family.

Kurt Alan Kitchen

==

I am a biochemist involved in AIDS-related viral research, as well as a mother. Being both a mother and a scientist can be very frustrating. So I have dedicated my quilt square to all the "AIDS babies" and made it from diapers and receiving blankets that were my own infant son's. The bottle, bibs, and toys attached to the square were all his. He is completely healthy—for which I am both thankful and slightly guilt-ridden. So many babies are not.

Science moves slowly. Patience is a necessity. But, please, know that we are doing the best that we can. The importance of our jobs does not go without note.

Sincerely,

Lisa M. Smith, Ph.D.

August 25, 1990

This quilt was made for Bernhard Lehmann. I loved him with all my heart and soul for 23 years, six months and 20 days. He was what I lived for. We had planned to die together because we wanted to die together as we had faced life together. But he could not wait for me and now I am lost without his love. I pray there is an afterlife so I can be with him again. I don't fear death anymore for I feel it will reunite me with Bernie.

. . . What I loved most about Bernie was his hands. He had big, masculine, rough, strong hands. And as strong and scrious as Bernie could be, you could touch his heart in an instant.

John Floda,
Lover and best friend of
Bernie Lehmann

May 18, 1990

It is truly difficult labor to tame and subdue hell and horror into a single expression of beauty . . .

I don't know why I chose all those crazy bubbles for the panel. It just happened that they came to be made. I wasn't planning it. But as I laid out the letters, phrases resurfaced to my thoughts; things he had said during his illness and during his last days in the hospital . . .

This is for my love, for my grief, for my letting go.

Cynthia was a very fragile, petite, Hispanic little girl whose mom is from El Salvador. When she was born, she had multiple medical problems, some of which required surgery and a blood transfusion. This is how she acquired AIDS.

She spent a lot of time in and out of hospitals. That's how we came to know her. Her mom was unable to care for her medical needs, so Cynthia was put into our foster home. She spoke about as much English as we did Spanish. Communication was often comical. She was an angel from above. Anyone that knew her would agree. Our families and friends accepted her with open arms. She was easygoing, patient, loving towards people and life.

Cynthia was in our home just a little over a year. We grew very close as a "family." When she left our home she went home to her mom. We maintained close contact for the remaining time she was in the world.

She is missed very much by a lot of people. However, we know she is with Jesus and is doing fine. She will always live in our memories and hearts. She was truly one of God's angels, sent to touch people's hearts and brighten their lives.

Roxie Mack and
Debra Argust

DUFF CHRISTOPHER PADDOCK

How does a mother find the words that can truly express her feelings about a beautiful human being that was her only son? He was stunningly handsome on the outside and equally lovely on the inside.

It has been a year since we lost our son, and his father and I are still grieving. The pain of losing him seems to worsen with time. We awaken each day and can't believe it all happened. How, where, when, why? No answers, just tears.

Duff was a person who, while alive, lived. We often shook our heads and said, "When is this boy going to get serious?" He was our little Peter Pan. Everybody loved him. The life of the party. He always stood out in a crowd. He was spoiled by his sister, and us, too, I guess, because we're a very sentimental type family.

Duff had finally made the big commitment to settle down, work hard, and become a success when this devastating disease attacked him. He had become a partner with his father, buying, building, and developing real estate. He could do anything. He would have been an enormous asset to the business as his taste and ideas were exceptional. This has been a heavy sadness for his father to carry, as their dreams together are a constant flashback that can never be realized. He lost his partner, his best friend, and his son. The first tract of homes has been completed without him. The joy, pleasure, and success of it was dwarfed by our loss and the reason for it all. In his memory, we named a street in the tract after him.

Duff and his sister had a wonderful relationship as brother and sister. He respected her so much. He was present at the birth of her first child, Aubree, now three. What a proud uncle he was. Our daughter gifted us with a second grandchild last July: a little boy who is named after his beloved uncle. His chosen name is Duff's middle name, Christopher.

I have pictures of our boy all over the house. Every Christmas and birthday, a new oil candle is added to a collection I have started in memory of him. An oil candle, picture, and the Quilt book sit on our coffee table in the living room. We miss him terribly.

When my thoughts for the panel started, I didn't know how or what to do. The design finally came to me because he loved Hawaii and the beautiful water so much. The palm tree seemed appropriate. The broken hearts represent our family. Two of the stars are in memory of two of his friends, Tom Bustamonte and Bill Lemon, who recently passed away of AIDS. We had taken care of our boy the last seven months of his life. This boy who loved life so much, and had so much to live for, never complained throughout this whole nightmare. The strength he displayed for us was so courageous. What a champion our son was.

When the end came, he was at home with us. It was the exact hour and moment that he was born: 8:46 p.m.

Donald L. and
Mary R. Paddock
(father and mother)

HOWARD Z. ROBINOWITZ ════════════

Howard I loved very much. Although it has now been four months since he died, only recently have I begun to let go. Ours was an intense relationship, short in duration. We met in a bereavement/healing group for people who had lost someone to AIDS or ARC. From the first time we met, he held a special place in my heart. We met in March 1986, and by September he was to enter the hospital and get a diagnosis of AIDS-related complex . . .

Howard was a lot to a lot of different people. To me, Howard was a good friend and someone I loved. And at times he was pure humor, lifting my spirits when they were really low.

One day, there were several friends in his bedroom as well as his nurse, and I was fussing about something he hadn't done. He looked at me and said, "You better be nice to me, I'm not going to be around much longer." You could hear everyone gasp for breath—they couldn't believe he had said that! I just laughed and told him guilt didn't work with me!

When Sandy and I made Howard's quilt, it was made as an act of love . . . With this quilt made and mailed, I will let him go. I hope he finds the peace that eluded him here on earth.

Love,
Rodney B. Holcomb

Dear Panel Maker,

My name is Randy Butts. Last week I worked at the NAMES Project showing in Birmingham. During that showing, thanks to a friend of mine, I came upon your panel for Timmy.

On behalf of myself and the rest of Timmy's family I would just like you to know how much it meant to us. It is comforting to know that there is someone out there that is that loving and thoughtful.

Please find enclosed a page including my name, address and phone number. I would really like it if you would please write me or phone me. I would really like it if I could thank you in person. It's important to me. I think Timmy would want it that way.

Looking forward to hearing from you.

Timmy's lover,

Randy Butts

Howard is sleeping in the buff. Well, actually, he's wearing a white t-shirt to give the appearance of being dressed to visitors. The police came and took him into custody. Later the State wouldn't let us see him. I decided that nothing would be gained or lost by dressing him. Then sealing him in two plastic body bags. So he sleeps eternally in a white t-shirt.

He died at home. With a cover over him, on the couch. At peace, with people he loved. We had had a hospital bed delivered the day before. But he just couldn't bring himself to lay on it. He said it made him cold. But in reality he had seen too much of that kind of thing in recent months.

He drifted in and out of sleep and consciousness for about two hours before he took his last breath. He would wake up, search the room until his eyes met mine, then drift off again. Once he said that it was making him tired to lay there and sleep. His Shanti pal called 911. I gave him mouth to mouth resuscitation. The lady on the phone told his Shanti pal how to do CPR. We put him down on the floor and tried to revive him until the rescue people arrived (which was very quick). No one could do anything. He was gone.

If you didn't know him, I'm a little sorry for you.
Because you missed knowing one of the really good
people. He was everyone's friend, and talked to
everyone he met, in line at the supermarket, walking
down the street, or sitting next to him in restaurants.
His needs were absolutely minimal. There were many
things he could not understand. Dishonesty was one of
them and he took great pride in his own honesty. Your
pleasure and happiness came before his own. His
innocence brought out the protective instincts in
everyone. On top of all this, he was really cute. He
had a way of smiling with his eyes that made you feel
special.

We have a double depth grave in Oak Hill
Cemetery. By universe time, I'll be in there with him
in the "wink of an eye." By the time the sun goes
supernova the concrete barrier between us will be dust
around us and we will be indistinguishable. Our
journey through eternity together will have just begun.

See ya soon lover!

Richard A. Kitterman

MAX PARKER

His full name was Ward Maxwell Parker, but he has always been called Max. He was born nine minutes before his twin sister, Anne, on February 16, 1963, at Fort Lewis in Tacoma, Washington. His father was a career Air Force doctor and pilot, his mother a good housewife and keeper of him and his three older brothers and twin sister.

As a youngster and throughout his life, he was soft-spoken and loving. He always wanted to be a part of whatever was going on at the time. He enjoyed helping people. He was an actor, dancer, singer, or model if one was needed.

One of Max's aunts spoke at his memorial service. Her words tell what we all feel about Max:

My nephew Max was a mascot. At Dobie Middle School in San Antonio, he was the first boy cheerleader the school ever had. His twin sister, Anne, played softball and his brothers were also on the playing fields. But Max was the star on the sidelines, leading the cheers. Max was a cheerleader.

To me, Max was a song. At the Organ Stop one night, when Grandmother and Granddaddy Harris were here, Max went up to the microphone and sang with the organ. We were sitting, eating our pizza, but

Max was in front of the crowd, singing "Edelweiss," a song about a noble white flower, blooming on the edge of the snow.

Max was like that flower. It's a white flower that blooms first in the spring. While the rest of us are here, huddled in the snow, Max is already out, blooming in the sunshine. Max was like a flower.

At the end, Max was a smile. When his body began to drift away and others had given up, Max would smile. Like a Cheshire cat, he faded away, but Max became a smile.

So while we go about our work on the playing field with the numbers on our backs, Max will be on the sidelines, cheering us on, singing a song, giving us a smile.

We will miss you, Max, for who among us doesn't need a cheerleader, a flower, a song, a smile?

Ray Wilson
(stepfather)
Rebecca Harris
(aunt)

Aaron Lee Sampson ══════════════

This panel for the AIDS Memorial Quilt honors the memory of Aaron Lee Sampson, 3-13-60 to 7-26-89.

Aaron was a great guy and I was lucky to have him as my lover for five years. Aaron was a simple man, he was happy with whatever he had. He had no big illusions of fame, or wealth, but just wanted the comfort of a home and lover. We had peace and we had love and now I'm lost.

The tears are already flowing as I write this. Words are so inadequate to express emotions. We were a great pair. We kept each other centered. Even our fights were fun.

Aaron loved to work. He had a job processing microfilm for a small firm. That was his worst day—when he had to come to the realization that he could not work anymore. He lost his focus. That was the beginning of the end.

We had a unique situation. As a registered nurse, I was able to take care of all his needs at home, except for a couple of hospitalizations. His insurance paid me to stay home so I was able to be with him always through his illness. We talked of death, but he made us focus on life. We came to the conclusion that after death there was something good out there, so there was no reason to be scared. We laughed, loved, and had fun until the last day.

Aaron loved me, cats and dogs, ice cream, county fairs, leather, sex, furniture and shopping. I'd want to go to the beach, he'd want to go to the furniture store to see what's new.

He would not like me trying to write about him. He was personal and private. He would say this was just between the two of us. And that's true. This is to help me. Aaron doesn't need help anymore. Aaron died with dignity. No pain and no regrets. I hope it's good for him out there.

Michael O. Murphy

We've lost our son. It is hard to believe that one in the prime of life is physically gone from us. Is it not supposed to be the older that depart from the living first? He brought to us the joys that always come to parents on being our firstborn. The one that will carry on the family name and its traditions. We grew with his successes and cried with him at his failures. We really didn't begin to know him until he came home in his manhood to spend his waning months with us. He left home at 18 and came back at 35, dying at 37. We are very grateful for this extra time we had with him.

He had his degree in communications and was so proud of that achievement, but he went back for graduate courses. He didn't want to give up. Also, he was striving to teach others to read. Always reading, studying to broaden his life. Always interested in a wide array of subjects; he knew his Roman and Greek history as well as their myths; art history and our language history and how it evolved. His love of nature helped him in his latter years with us; this helped him hold fast to his faith in God.

He was a teacher, teaching me not to judge lest we be judged. He taught us compassion even though he was in a no-win situation. He taught us to love each other, make each day count for it might be our last. Even in his darkest hours he brought our family, more than ever, closer together. Indeed, he was a teacher, probably my best.

Is he gone? Yes, but as it is written, "Those we love are with the Lord, and the Lord has promised to be with us. If they are with Him, and He is with us . . . they cannot be far away." He will be sorely missed.

This memorial to our son gives us great pleasure, and we present it to you with grateful hearts.

Mr. and Mrs. R.M.K.

Col. Kenneth J. Wittenberg

He was U.S. Army Colonel Kenneth J. Wittenberg, 53 years old . . . my lover, my brother, my father, my son, my best friend for 17 years. When you are together for 17 years, you go through a lot of phases. Kenneth and I met while I was still in the Army . . . he was a Major and I was a Sergeant.

He was the most straight-arrow, tight-assed, disciplined, no-nonsense, hard-headed kind of guy you could ever meet. I was a crazy guy in the theatre business, praying to get out of the Army. At first glance, we are not talking a match made in heaven. But we took care of each other and nurtured our love for 17 years.

He taught me how to keep my checkbook balanced, how to be a man, how to take responsibility for myself and how to love. I taught him how to have a good time, how to take himself a lot less seriously and how to love.

Kenneth found he had AIDS shortly after his retirement from the Army . . . with 30 years service.

We had made and kept many very close friends over the years who were all there for him and me when he became ill. The amazing part of the whole tragic mess was how he transformed all of us with his integrity and love in the dying process. He made the experience spiritual for his family, my family and our wonderful friends. He was at Walter Reed Army Medical Center for his illness. The staff at that hospital should all be canonized. Kenneth transformed them, too.

continued

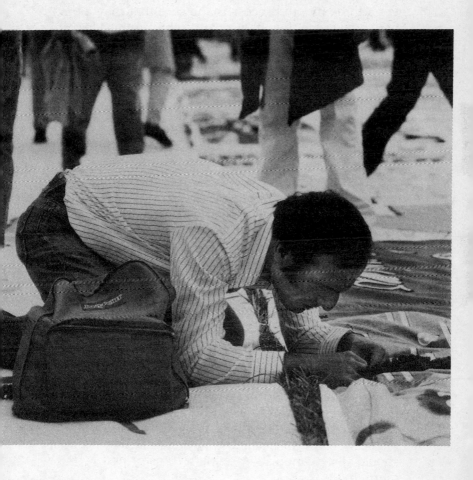

Col. Kenneth J. Wittenberg

He wanted to die at home. His will and personal affairs were in impeccable order, of course. Then he methodically summoned all those he had loved, and over a three month process made sure that they all knew how much they had meant to him in his life. When he was done he told me to take him home because he was ready to die. He died at home holding my hand as I read him poetry . . . just like he had wanted.

Three days before he died, he struggled for 10 minutes to communicate his last words: "When I die, I want everyone to get together and have a wonderful time."

He had more medals, awards, plaques and things than you can possibly imagine. He was an incredible athlete. He had courage, integrity and commitment which should humble us all. And his final gift to us was the exemplary manner in which he died . . . selfless, loving and with a little sense of ironic humor.

It was later we learned the number of charities he had contributed to for years . . . Korean orphans, animals, the opera, etc. There were so many we had to write a form letter to send them.

God, how I loved that man.

Bless you all,

Kary M. Walker

My dearest Bob,

There is not a word to describe how much I miss you, much more than I ever realized I would. I miss not being able to talk to you because you always understood and you always made everything seem better. I really, really miss your sense of humor, your ability to express something comical.

The jokes that you could tell and then your laugh—I can still hear it. How I so enjoyed that funny little poem you and only you could recite; how I had always wanted you to record it for me, or I was going to and somehow it was never done and I am so sorry I didn't. I miss not having you to watch the 'skin games with and how excited you got just watching how excited I got, and I'll never part with the Redskin puppet you gave me. I miss being able to call you to fix or do something for me or to go shopping with me. When I hear a song you really liked and listening to certain songs you and Darlene danced so well to . . . I miss doing things for you and trying to make you feel better, and I miss sitting on your bed and our talks just before you went to sleep, and I miss holding your hand so it would not shake. I just miss everything about you.

When you died, I wanted to die. I kissed and held you and I hope you heard me say, "I love you." I didn't believe it at first, and I felt so numb, and all I could think was "It's over, and I didn't want it to be this way." I came home and even though there were family and friends here, the house seemed so empty and all I could think was, you would never be back

continued

here and you would not be here for me to take care of. I just despise being in this house and I go out most days, but the evenings are so long and there is really nowhere I want to go alone. I hate the weekends, too, but I can find something to do, usually. I miss not being able to take you to the mall, or just for a ride.

Bob, I am so lonely for you. Not a day goes by that I don't cry. So many, many things make me think of you. It seems like it gets worse instead of better. I keep thinking the next day will be better and I think of so many things that need to and should be done, but I have no desire to do them. I am in the car driving somewhere, and all of a sudden the tears roll down my face. It's the same in the grocery store or in the mall. I hold your picture and can almost feel you. I wonder if I will ever feel like having a good time or laughing again, or will there ever be happiness in this house again, and will we ever have another party with dancing and singing and a good time?

I don't think there was anything we did not talk about or discuss and I don't think there was anything ever said to hurt either one. I'm so glad you were here, so I could tell you how much I loved you every day and every night before you went to bed. To tell you what a wonderful son you had been all your life, and how very proud I was and still am. I have not one thing to be ashamed of, and I know you did not.

I wish I could have prevented your illness—God knows I would have given my life for you. I wish I could "kiss it all better" like I used to do when you were a little boy and make it go away. Somehow it was in the hands of God. When you were born a "blue baby" He let you live through it and it may have been too much to ask for a second chance, even though I tried. I really, truly feel I did everything I could to make this last year as comfortable for you as possible. I'm angry at myself that there was absolutely not one thing in this world that I could do to save your life. I can never describe the totally helpless feeling I suffered each day . . .

I only ask that you save a place for me for the day I will see you again. Help me make it through all the days and nights till then.

Bob, you and I had a wonderful relationship, and I would just pray that more mothers and sons could enjoy each other as much. I felt so proud when you would take me to the clubs and you seemed so proud of me and we had so much fun and laughed and danced, and I'm so happy to tell you what a pleasure it has been to have a son who could also be a best friend.

Right now, I am not happy about anything going on in my life. The only happiness I have had, if you can call it that, is when you passed away. I had told you your arm and hand would not shake anymore, you would be able to walk and dance once again, your eyesight would be good again, your speech would become normal again. There would be peace, contentment, and sunshine every day and you would

continued

be in a far better place. And even though you are gone, I just know you are happy and that's all that really matters. I will see you again, my friend, my son.

Your loving mother,
Ruth M. Eshmont

November 1, 1988

P.S.: I visit your grave several times a week. On your birthday I took some very beautiful peonies and balloons. One balloon was white and in red it said, "I love you," the other had a big pumpkin with Snoopy in it. The other day I took another balloon and stuck it in the flowers. Guess what? It had the Redskin helmet on it—thought you would like that even though they played a horrible game this weekend. I ordered your marker and you would be proud of me. It will be beautiful. It has a vase for flowers which I keep there all the time. Under that I had an inscription engraved: "Courage in the face of fear," then your name and the dates, and in between the dates, an Air Force insignia. Love ya!

Sammy De Marco was a much nicer person than you will hear from me. Others found him loving, sweet-natured, gentle, etc. I knew him as an aggravation, dependent on his ex-lover, Lewis Love (my own sweetheart, who died a month after Sam, and whose panel should be received in the same batch, I imagine).

As much as I would like to detail my resentments, let me release and heal them with this panel. Lewis loved Sam dearly, and as he is also dead, I have done what he would have done to honor Sam. In keeping honest with my impression and experience of knowing him, I have kept this as simple as I could. Plain brown background, simple black letters. Sam had beautiful bronze skin and black hair. The blue heart and spikes going through it are for his pained existence. It's a shame he lost so much of his life to drug abuse. The small heart within is for Lewis, the one hard and fast love he always had for his own, yet could never recognize through his own floundering. I added the photo, showing silhouettes of Sam and Lewis when they were lovers.

There is proof that he was loved.

I have an old phone book of Lewis's, where he recorded all friends and acquaintances and romantic partners. By many names were short descriptions to remind him who the people were. There would be a name, and address or phone number, and "Great!" or "HOT" or "Gorgeous" . . . but Sammy's name was followed without address or number, just simply the word: "GOD."

Ross MacLean

I didn't know David. He was the next-door-neighbor of my lover Lisa and her family in Moorhead. He died in the winter of '87–'88. I just wanted to make a panel for him so he would be remembered, even if it only be through my imagination.

She said he was a biologist who loved flowers and all of the wonders of nature really. So the panel has pictures of some of the things that he might have seen and known on the prairie—the birdsfoot violet (*viola pidata*), the meadowlark, the brilliant sun, a prairie windmill and prairie dogs kissing. She also said he used to wear jeans and a tee shirt a lot, so I can imagine him tying a bandanna around his neck once in a while just to be fancy.

It has felt good to me to be able to stand up in the middle of this sad time and be able to make this memorial. I don't personally know anyone who's died of AIDS, but I think I am, in a way, preparing myself for the eventuality, and this has helped.

I hope my spiritual friend likes his quilt. It's stuffed with goose down, and in a pinch I think it could even keep him warm against the winter prairie winds.

Alice Erickson

July 12, 1988

Peter Deaett was brilliant.

He would have laughed at hearing himself described as such. But I could easily gather an extensive list of names of people who would attest whole-heartedly to the appropriateness of such praise. Peter was like no one else. An original. A self-made man.

Peter was not college-educated, he was not a big reader of books and his vocabulary was short on multi-syllable words. He was extremely self-effacing and rather insecure about his intelligence. But his mind and wit were quicker and livelier than anyone I've ever known. Peter grew up in Southern California—a region that would irreversibly effect his unique aesthetic. His vision was filled with desert, trailer parks, California pottery, cowboy boots and dope. In these areas and more, Peter was an expert.

He owned what is perhaps the world's best and most extensive collection of paint-by-numbers. He was an accomplished photographer and his work consisted of the subjects that made up the constellation of his obesssions—cemeteries, old gas pumps, trailers, found objets d'art.

As defined by his obesssions as Peter was, it would be a misconception to perceive him as being materialistic. His things came to him and just as easily he sent them back out into the world. Peter could have authored a book titled, "Zen and the Art of Garage Sales."

continued

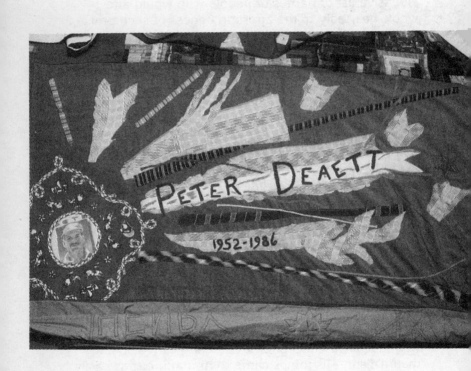

PETER DEAETT

1952-1986

He was a master, and I am his disciple. An active thrifting addict, I am always very conscious of Peter sitting on my shoulder, directing my eye, urging me to look a little closer at a seemingly worthless pile of junk for the hidden treasure, whispering hope into my ear as I approach yet another Salvation Army store . . . in this way and more he is with me always.

Michael Baum

I lost my lover, Gary Dicovich, on April 28, 1990, after being together for over six years. His two year battle with AIDS just seems to add one more victim to the body count because of public and government apathy toward the AIDS crisis.

I decided to make a panel for the Quilt after feeling so helpless in the awareness battle for AIDS. It's sad that we have to make these panels at all, but hopefully the sheer number of panels and the lost lives that they represent will have some kind of impact on the general public.

Gary was cremated and scattered without a permanent memorial stone, so the quilt panel is also my way of immortalizing him, at least as long as the fabric holds up. I hoped I would never have to make him a panel, but now that he's gone I feel that it is important to give him a memorial for all of the pain that he's endured. To a certain extent, the panel is also for me. All of the pain and loss that I've gone through to be by his side through this horrible ordeal.

Three of our friends, Bud Beatty, Karen Ames and Valerie Lynn, helped me make the panel. It was our first time sewing anything, and I'm glad that it was such a loving, heartfelt project.

David Bender

July 20, 1990

Billy Denver Donald was my brother. He was born in Dorsey, Michigan on June 18, 1936—he died April 23, 1987.

Physically, he was tall with black hair, blue eyes and olive complexion—exceptionally handsome. He was a father to a 19-year-old son, a brother to three sisters, a son to a widowed mother, a special nephew to many aunts and uncles, a cousin to about 60, a friend, a highly respected manager to his fellow workers, and so much more.

I was sitting in the hospital waiting room after just being told Bill had AIDS. I mentally became very small—lifted off the sofa—went out the window and landed on the grass. The wind blew a leaf over me and I hid from the world for a few seconds.

With God's help and Bill's courage, we dealt with his illness with all the love within us. And life goes on without him. We will miss him forever.

Norma Shumpert
Sister of Billy Denver Donald

September 14, 1987

Debbie Lynn Karr was born in Tulsa on May 1st, 1957. She remained in Tulsa until her adult years and then began to travel. Debbie was a gourmet cook and used fresh herbs while preparing her favorite meals. She loved all of nature's animals, flowers and birds. She always had pets; her last pet was a black chow named Kadi. During her life she lived in many states from the west coast to the east coast. She was married in Waco, Texas, then moved to Tucson, Arizona, where her daughter Katrina Kay was born.

Debbie became ill and was misdiagnosed for over a year. She was diagnosed with AIDS in July of 1989. The disease had progressed to a point that it was difficult to keep it under control.

Debbie wrote the following note a few weeks before she was admitted to the hospital for the last time:

To Those Concerned:
It's funny how things begin to fit together when you look back in retrospect. I am a 33-year-old single mother with a beautiful six-year-old little girl. I was diagnosed almost a year ago with AIDS.
It's hard to explain the fear, guilt and anxiety you feel when you are faced with a

terminal illness. With AIDS there are so many social prejudices you have to deal with as well as the physical problems you have.

I live in a small town and I'm not able to be up-front with anyone about my illness. It's not necessarily that I can't handle the rejection, but I worry about my daughter. People can be so cruel.

It's not as if you could contract AIDS through casual contact. There are only two ways you can get AIDS—from sex and from blood. Mine was caused by two units of blood I received following surgery. This was in January of 1985. Unfortunately, screening of blood for the AIDS virus did not begin until March of that year. I always seem to be a day late and a dollar short.

Debbie Karr

Debbie lived until 7 p.m., September 24, 1990. She was dearly loved and will be missed by her daughter, Katrina, her puppy Kadi, her mother, dad, brothers and her many friends.

Debbie's Mom

REVELLE DAVIS, JR. ═══════════════

This panel was created as a tribute to Revelle L. Davis, Jr. by his mother, Virginia James and his AIDS Project Los Angeles buddy, Sue Sprowls; his friend, Richard Chuvala, assembled, packaged and shipped the panel to the NAMES Project.

In creating the panel, we used as our guides the poem which is embroidered on the quilt, and the memorial service which was held for Revelle on April 30th. Shortly after Revelle's death, Virginia found the poem in Revelle's journal. The poem expresses the childlike faith which Revelle confessed.

Revelle could be rough and gruff but when it came to the things he loved most dearly, there was a sweet innocence in his approach to life. He spoke of caring for his nephew, whom he adored. He talked of wanting to find a husband for his mother, so she would have someone to care for her.

Revelle could yell and demand with the best of them, but he would also greet me quietly in the hospital, saying "I felt like crying earlier but I wanted to wait until you were here; I feel I can cry with you." An hour later, he'd slide into a chair with me and burst into the tears he'd been saving for my visit.

Making the panel was a project of love and remembrance, full of all that was Revelle. Virginia and I stood in the fabric store one day, trying to decide between two bolts of blue fabric for the background: which one more closely represented the blue of the sky? We excused ourselves for a moment and walked outside to look at the sky. Between us, Virginia and I have many experiences looking at the sky and would normally have had no problem choosing a "pale blue" sky. But as I said to her with a laugh as we stood on the sidewalk, fabric in hand, looking toward the heavens, "Only Revelle could make us feel insecure about the color of the sky!" We joked that we could hear him laughing at us for being so "foolish" as not to know what color he meant when he wrote "pale blue."

Knowing Revelle, caring for Revelle, loving Revelle—meant learning about unconditional love. It meant loving someone who lumbered down the hospital corridor to the lounge, dragging his IV behind him, screaming at the top of his lungs, provoking tears to flow from your eyes—and then turned and asked for a hug. Loving Revelle meant finding the humor in his demanding nature. One night, when we were chiding him about how well we cared for him, he said, "Yeah, you guys are really good to me, but you know what? With all I'm going through, I think I deserve it." This comment instantly earned him the nickname "Prince Revelle."

Revelle was self-motivated, independent. He hated the dependency that came with the advanced stages of his illness. He was not, ultimately, able to express it with more than his presence, but there was no question that all the energy and anger that drove him throughout his life continued to drive him at the end. Revelle did not go gentle into that good night.

Susan F. Sprowls

July 29, 1988

The enclosed quilt is in memory of our dear son, Gary L. We have described him on the quilt as he was—loving, loved, talented, witty, generous . . . He was a bright light in our lives that is now dark.

We have wonderful memories of his life—his life which was one of our greatest gifts. We wish we could hug him and say "we love you" again, but since we can't we are sending and sharing this quilt of love.

Thank you for starting the NAMES Project and for all of you—good health—and COURAGE.

Love,

Midwesterner

August 8, 1988

The history of Project NAAM-Chewit (which means, in essence, "life-names") started in a hospital outside Bangkok, where most people with HIV and AIDS are receiving treatment. We showed videos to the people there, mostly entertainment, music or something fun and one was the Quilt display which was a contribution from the NAMES Project. That was around August 1989. Every time we visited the hospital, we met relatives or friends of those who are being treated there. We talked with them and made some friends. We did not really know what we were heading for, but only desired to be friends with people who do not want to be seen in public, or even have their story told to anyone, only because they have or are related to those who have AIDS.

We met Panya, a PWA who was a semi-pro soccer player, still waiting to have his joint-losing upper leg bone put back in place, after five refusals from different hospitals in Bangkok. And he kept trying and trying . . .

Another person was Pramote, a homeless man being cured for his drug habit. Both Panya and Pramote had become close friends there. Pramote helped Panya with washing his body, took him to the toilet, as well as tirelessly doing services for everyone in the ward.

At that time we were also preparing a free open-air concert in the park to raise funds for our work with people living with AIDS. The event was held on January 22, 1990, and it was overwhelmed with about 40,000 people and was broadcast live on national TV. The objective of this event was to encourage PWAs to regain their confidence and will to live. It was

continued

also our hope to reduce social prejudice and mis-conceptions about people with AIDS.

We helped Panya to petition the Ministry of Health. Finally, after a four-month press campaign, one government hospital took him. It was eight months later, after a press followup campaign, that Panya was admitted to the hospital for his leg operation in December 1990.

During that time, we (including Panya and Pramote) decided to make World AIDS Day cards and sent them to the Prime Minister, as well as ministers and high officers in the Public Health Ministry. We also sent them to doctors and nurses who took good care of them and other people whom they wished to send them to. Panya and Pramote were the organizing forces behind this good wishes campaign.

In March 1991, Panya was out of the hospital. We did not claim the success of getting Panya into the operating room, but somehow the whole campaign had shown our strength. Especially Panya and Pramote felt their power and were determined to work in support of other people with HIV.

Panya and Pramote helped us compile lists of their friends, whom they met while in the hospital. They contacted those families, told them that we wanted to make memorial quilts for their loved ones and asked them about some personal information on those who were to be remembered. Most people agreed with what we wanted to do, but when asked to join us in making the quilts, they felt uncomfortable about participating and allowed us to make quilts for them instead.

Panya could not go with us to the northeast, as he still needed to see the doctor after his leg operation. Pramote was left behind to look after him. Something must have been going on in his mind throughout that time. He must have felt lonely and had no hope in the continuation of his homeless life. We came back to Bangkok, feeling that we had really started something. The next day, we heard that Pramote was put back in the hospital. Shortly thereafter, he ran away and started to take drugs again. When he came back, he was very weak and very quiet. We did not really realize how serious his condition was. Pramote died in the hospital two weeks later. It was Saturday, June 21, 1991. That day we held another party at the hospital which we all had planned together. Though the party went well, it was very hard for all of us to accept it as a memorial gathering to Pramote. It was a very quiet one.

Pramote had decided to take his own life before AIDS would. His funeral was held the next day. It was only eight of us and two monks who led the ceremony. We are still searching for his relatives. We always think of Pramote and feel that he is still around with us. We have our 49th quilt with Pramote's name on it. November 1991 is our one-year anniversary and we will dedicate this to him.

. . . It has been a good year for us, so far. And when we look ahead, we see more people seeking friendship and many friends passing away with memories to remember. The reality is that many quilts will be made and displayed. Recognitions may count the effects of our work. But we do not want only that. Remembering people who died is more important, for people who live to learn. And that is when we do not have to make and display quilts any more.

Chumpon Apisuk
NAAM-Chewit, Thailand

Dear Garry,

I remember the first time we met. I did your intake at the clinic. I was struck by your openness. I had no idea we would become such friends.

It took another year before our friendship developed. I had quit my job—you offered me a job cleaning—I declined. When you came to my apartment you understood why. You were so supportive during the AIDS Mastery. It was your job to give everyone their medication at the right time. I liked not having to think about it.

That summer we drove up with three other people to Minneapolis for a very intense seminar. I'll never forget the ride back to Chicago. Such strange things happened. We spoke of life after death. You said you wanted to be Shirley MacLaine in your next life. We all spoke so openly during that car ride. You told me that if you died before me you would send me a sign to prove there was life after death. A pair of black fishnet stockings. It's been four months, Garry! I'm still waiting!

Last summer, you and Jose came to Navy Pier, where I was volunteering with the Quilt. I took a break and Jose pushed you in the wheelchair while I walked beside you looking at all the panels. We cried at Brian Hamilton's and that's when you told me you wanted your panel to say "Diagnosed ? years and they were damn good."

I hope you would like the way I made it. I'm sure you would have some smart remark to say like "Not bad for a straight woman!"

God, Garry, I miss you so much.

Where the hell are those fishnets?

Love,
Andrea S. Gerson

First of all I would like to begin by saying that writing about Brett and his life is so very, very hard.

My life was never the same from the moment I met him 10 years ago, and my life will never be the same until we meet again.

I met Brett at the airport; he worked for Budget Rent A Car at the time, I worked for Avis. From the moment we met there was an instant bond that comes when you truly find someone who is going to be a very special person in your life. Brett could be described as an Armani suit, a laugh and a smile that could brighten anyone's darkened corner. God how I miss him.

Brett had just moved here from New York one year prior to me meeting him. I myself was born and raised in the Bay Area. It's so very strange to just say "Marilyn" now, because to all our friends "Brett and Marilyn" was just one word. About one year or so after our meeting we moved in together. Oh, the times we had going to Mexico, L.A., watching "Golden Girls" and laughing; oh how his laughter made you feel so good.

As time went on the virus began to eat at him. It

was getting close to the holidays so I asked him if he would like to go home—back east. He was so happy. Brett's favorite time of the year was Christmas. He comes from a large family—three sisters and two brothers.

He left San Francisco on November 22, 1989 with the expectation of returning after the first of the new year. Brett began regressing rapidly and came down with tuberculosis. The last time I spoke to him was December 28, 1989. He died at home on New Year's Day in the middle of the night. Words are just not enough to describe when his mom called with the news. I flew back to New York the next day. His service was beautiful. As it was so close to Christmas, all the holiday things were still glowing, just as he always was.

His closest friends and I have made this quilt as a tribute to him. God, he would have only been 30 years old this year. Because of this horrible disease his *puzzle* was never fully completed. I know he is at peace, but we will all be at peace only when this dreadful disease is stopped and a cure is found. *PLEASE* let it be soon.

Marilyn Navilhon

Benjamin L. Santiago was a brave, intelligent, generous, and very good-looking person. I loved and took care of him until the very end of his mortal life. Nothing would stop me! I even gave up my job to be with him! In our 12 short years together, we lived, loved and learned from each other, and I miss him with all my heart and soul!

Those people who have not been through the experience of watching a healthy young person slowly and painfully die before their eyes will never be able to truly understand; they just honestly can't relate.

Unfortunately I had to keep the secret of his illness from many friends and relatives because of the ignorance and narrow-mindedness that presently exists. These people were not mean or cruel individuals. They just would not understand—they had not experienced it!

As a Public Health Educator, my main mission in life is to educate as many people as possible about this devastating but preventable disease.

My wish is that people help themselves to become more educated, knowledgeable, open-minded, loving and compassionate to those who have AIDS. So that people as myself and others, who suffered extremely, don't go through the agony alone!

People who have AIDS have nothing to be ashamed of. They are strong and brave souls. God bless them all!

Yours in health,

Denise Santiago-Rodriguez

Prostitute with AIDS dies from the disease—
United Press International
HOLLYWOOD, FLA.—[W.A.B.], who worked as a
prostitute knowing she had AIDS, died from
complications of the disease Saturday at
Memorial Hospital while serving a four-year
prison sentence for arson. She was 20.

B. had been arrested 17 times in Dade
County for prostitution. She once said in court
she did not tell her customers she had acquired
immune deficiency syndrome unless "they look
like they can handle it."

"I know I should tell my tricks to use
condoms," she told the *Miami Herald* last year,
"but a lot of them don't want to and if they
don't want to, I'm still going to date them
because business is business."

Ms. B. said she performed sexual acts with
hundreds of men to support her drug habit. She
believed she got the AIDS virus while injecting
drugs.

I read this in the *Boston Globe* and made this
panel. She is the same age as my granddaughter (who
will graduate from MIT next June!).

W.A. needed my panel—and I needed to do it!

Anne W. Luedeman

My dearest Steven:

I miss you so much. It's hard to get up some mornings, knowing that I won't see your face.

We shared so many things together besides this virus. Our thoughts sometimes scared us because we would both say the same thing at the same time.

I was so glad I was able to be with you and they allowed me to spend time with you after you passed on to your new life.

I can't stop the tears from flowing and the emptiness in my heart still hurts. But I know that you are with me in my heart and soul. Every trip I get to take you are with me. Oh, I almost forgot. I went to a Cubs game. I never got to go with you.

This quilt is the show of my love to you. The love of baseball is shown by your jacket. The love for your cat and the red rose is love you showed for life. Finally your picture with the stained glass window you and I painted shows our love we shared.

Please give me strength and hope. I still need it and feel it each time I look at your picture.

Till we are united again.
All my love,

John J. Bahr

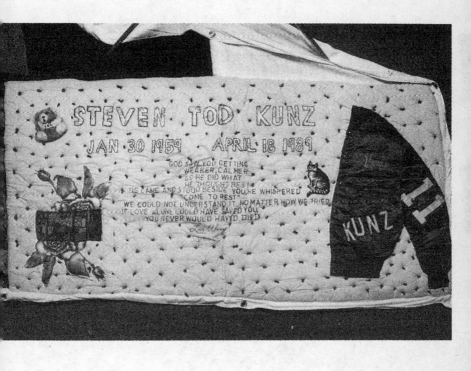

Dear Kirk,

A lot has happened since you passed. Bush got elected President. Dan is seeing someone and romance may even be stalking me.

I made a panel for you—I wanted it to be representative of your many interests and talents, but a lot is symbolic as I discovered that my skills as a quilter could be better. I chose a background piece of fabric that was a lot like the English imitation Chinese wallpapers of the 1760s because it reminded me of your travels to Europe, your interest in cooking and music, and your ability to write such clear and direct prose. The cloth had an 18th-century flavor to it, and so did you—wonderfully well-rounded and talented in so many areas.

I could have made block letters for your name, but somehow it would not have been you. Instead, I rounded the edges, elongated them a bit and curved your name across the top. This symbolized to me your willingness to reach out and explore, as well as that flexibility one needs to enjoy life fully. I marked out the letters in magic marker, and left the marker intact—it symbolizes to me the fact that you weren't finished having a good time with us when you left us.

"Too Good" speaks for itself. I did it differently, almost hurriedly, in magic marker on a piece of sheet to emphasize how fleeting words are, but yet that they may possess an unexpected permanence. I am no quilter, however, and at this point "Too Good" is askew under your name. I've asked the NAMES Project to center it below your name and I hope that they will do so.

It was hard to give up your panel to the NAMES Project. I think of you often. Be your own gracious, sweet self.

Your friend,

Jeff Kilpatrick

August 30, 1989

David Bell was kind of the John Hancock of PWAs in Chicago. He was very active in advocating for the rights of PWAs and together David and I helped to start the Chicago chapter of NAPWA.

David was a strong person and very outspoken. He wanted to be remembered for his activism. Not everyone liked him. It was felt that he was a publicity hound. David had articles written about him in all of the Chicago newspapers and in several national magazines. He was very proud of the fact that he was getting to be well known.

I think David was the kind of person you either loved or hated. I loved him.

He was so big! Over 6 feet tall (several inches) and husky. It was hard to believe he was sick. I didn't always believe him when he complained of pain. Sometimes I felt he just wanted the attention.

February 14, 1988, David married John Tudor in the Unitarian Church. It was the first gay wedding I had ever been to. David's parents Laurel and Gerry gave him away. David was very fortunate having the parents he had. They were supportive of everything he did.

David was a generous person. He would frequently buy gifts for his friends. One day David asked me to try on the new leather jacket he was wearing. I did and he said "Just as I thought. It looks better on you than on me. You can have it after I die." About a month before he died, David handed me the jacket while I was visiting. I went into my car with it and screamed and screamed. I couldn't imagine life without him around!

When I decided to become a foster parent, David was the most supportive of my friends. It saddens me that he died before my foster daughter came to live with me. He would have liked her.

While making his panel I burned myself several times with the glue gun and I just know that wherever he is, David laughed and said "I'm worth it!"

Andrea

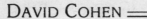

We took care of our friend, wonderful, flashy, crazy David Cohen.

Hope there are enough sequins.

We love you, David.

Bob Vogel,
Susan Shaw,
John Roberto,
Paula Chiotti

September 15, 1987

I have lost someone dear to me to AIDS. My husband.

It is too late for me to participate. If possible, maybe you could stencil "F.T." in a corner—I will be watching your accomplishments.

Good luck, A.T.

The reason I do not want anyone to know (including my children) is because no one except his doctor and I know. Thank you.

Vinnie was a friend of mine for about 10 years—off and on we fought and laughed. I hadn't seen him for about five years.

Vinnie was an Italian man who loved to cook and always had a beautiful house. Vinnie found me my first house when I had my first child—whenever she would cry he would say "give her some raisins and hold her till she stops." Vinnie loved elephants—he had so many in his collection.

I got to spend time with Vinnie again. His last weeks on earth we talked about old times and lost time. He told me he loved me. I'll never forget it. He talked to his father a few days before he died. That was very special to him.

That baby he used to hold is now 10 years old—Starbright is her name—she made this banner all by herself—Vinnie gave her his elephant, which she calls Vinnie and loves very much.

Thank you, Vinnie,

Betsy Bilyck and
Starbright Bilyck

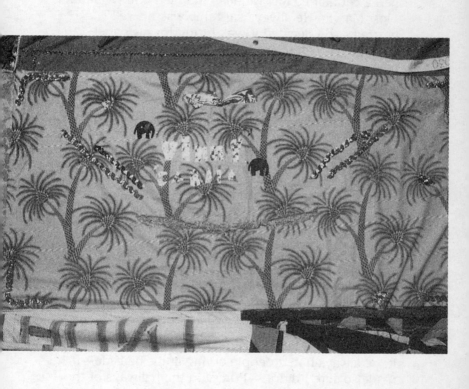

This is a copy of a postcard Marvin sent to me in December 1985, ten months before he died. He'd already had his first bout of pneumocystis and was regaining his strength. He had a cat named Evelyn; I had a cat named Ms. Kiques. She died one week after I lost Marvin. He always said this was his self-portrait—so I decided it was fitting for his panel. I think he's up there laughing at the fact that it's a picture of a nice Asian man with the unlikely name of a nice Jewish boy.

Marvin laughed a lot, but he always had this . . . edge to him. Sort of a fiery anger. No, not anger really—more of an impatience with the rest of the world. He was very bright—very attuned to refinement, perfection and beauty in the world. He could be so passionate about a scene from a play, or an antique kimono or the taste of a wine. But it was almost as if he'd known all along he hadn't much time—he moved at a fast pace and required that the rest of the world be sharp and move along with him. And if it didn't he didn't have time for it.

That intensity threw me sometimes—and it also drew me to him. He was fiercely loyal and so observant and supportive of those he loved. He even snuggled hard.

Now as I write of his death, I start to cry—damn it, he always hated people crying at his bedside—I made so sure I didn't—I'd cry in the hallways of the hospital, I'd cry just outside his room, I'd cry as I tried to sleep in the room in his parents' house the week before he died—listening to Marvin coughing in the room to my left and his parents weeping for him in

continued

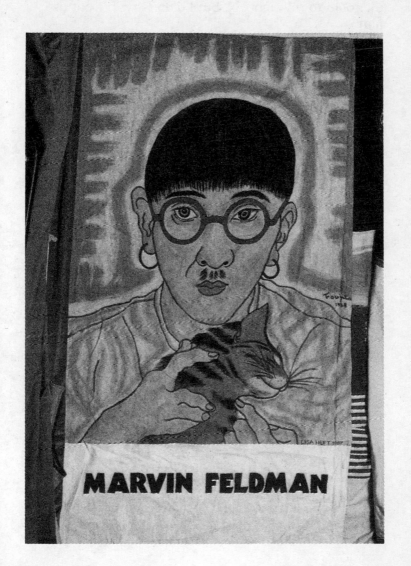

MARVIN FELDMAN

the room to my right . . . But I didn't cry in front of him.

We'd talk, we'd watch TV, we'd take medication and we'd eat "Jell-o Jewels," as he bravely endured all the pain and frustration. He didn't have much energy left for being angry, so we talked and talked and talked. He told me what it felt like when he'd decided that he didn't have to fight anymore, that it was OK to die. He still had that fierceness left to him, though—I remember him refusing to be carried to the bathroom when he could no longer walk—he crawled down the hall . . . his father carried him back.

I told him I was going to celebrate his passing by opening a bottle of champagne somewhere pretty like Golden Gate Park—he said, "You know, Lees—I never really liked champagne . . ."

Damn him, he was going to orchestrate his very own memorial service. And so he did. For his funeral, a simple casket with five white roses laid down on it— for his memorial a week later five of us went out to Land's End and tossed white roses into the surf and drank his favorite sauvignon blanc.

Lisa Heft

September 1987

Roy Cohn was a horrible human being. During the 1950s Cohn served as right-hand-man for Sen. Joseph McCarthy's Communist and anti-gay witchhunts. Cohn's vicious tactics and innuendo ruined hundreds of lives, and drove who knows how many to desperation and suicide. After the country rightfully saw fit to take away McCarthy's ill-used power, Cohn became legendary as probably the shiftiest lawyer in the country.

Always in the public eye, Cohn was questioned on many occasions about the allegations of his homosexuality. The allegation was always completely refuted. Even after he was hospitalized Cohn denied his homosexuality and claimed his illness to be a liver disease. His medication and hospital records indicated AIDS.

Many people would argue that a shallow grave and a handful of lime would be a fitting tribute to the legacy of Roy Cohn. Many would argue that living a closeted life is one thing, but ruining other lives with a zeal that can only be described as sadistic is unforgivable. And they're right.

But Roy Cohn died of AIDS. And whether you liked him or hated him, the fact remains that Roy Cohn died of AIDS. He was ashamed to be gay, and I'm ashamed that he was one of us. He was a bully, yes. A coward, yes. He was also a victim of this horrible disease.

Paul McCarthy

Maria died when she was only four years old. Neither she nor anyone else knew why at the time. It was several years after her death that it was discovered that she had died of AIDS.

Maria was a remarkable child. All who knew her were affected by her. She was beautiful, sweet, and beguiling. She had a powerful presence. Even though she never learned to speak, she had a wisdom about her that showed in her eyes and was sometimes disconcerting in someone so young.

Born three months prematurely, Maria was off to a rough start. Her mother, Elizabeth, apparently had AIDS at the time of Maria's birth. (She has since died of the disease.) In retrospect, Maria's illness and its progression were classic, a study in pediatric AIDS. But at the time, she was an enigma. It was obvious that she had a disorder of her immune system, but none of the specialists could figure it out.

I met Maria when she was two years old and in the hospital with pneumonia. I was one of the nurses involved in her care, and, for a variety of reasons (one of which was her homelessness, neither of her parents was able to care for her); I took her home with me as my foster daughter. She lived with me for a year. During that time, I watched her grow from a withdrawn, very ill child to a delightful, responsive, loving, almost healthy child. Her health ultimately failed, but perhaps it was best that no one knew of this inevitability.

We treated her like a normal child. She loved to go for walks in her stroller, taking in everything around her, and for some reason was thrilled by the pigeons on 24th Street. She loved Naked Hour, that time at the end of the day when changing into her pajamas: she would scream with laughter when tickled or when Martha the cat rubbed against her legs. She understood everything that was said to her, and somehow managed to make her desires known without using words. She was an incorrigible flirt, and won the hearts of everyone who knew her.

Maria had a spirit that transcended the frustrations and pain to which she was subjected. She left those who knew her feeling blessed for having been a part of her life.

Julie Simon

Dear Charley,

Is it just four days ago that you died, leaving behind those images that keep me from sleep? I am so sad, Charley. I don't grieve for your life, which was magical. You described paradise when you spoke of growing up: shell-hunting all summer on Pawley's Island; waiting out, in the hammock, the afternoon thunderstorms; letting the waves roll you to shore. Rusty and DaDa remember. Baylis and Kit remember. Your mama can't forget.

How many in [Charleston] remember? I don't know half their names. They know yours—Cholly Holly, Cholly Holly—and speak it to call up by incantation, life, fun, a sense of themselves. Do they, like me, feel they can be themselves only around you? If so, we must look for ourselves in memory.

Strangers call me to make some connection. Over long distance, each voice is a cry: "This loss is MINE." Kathy remembers, Gina and Cletus remember—maybe Gina remembers most.

The last 14 years are mine, and now they ask me to write something about "how you should be remembered." I wish that just one of us could remember you right, exactly as you were, because then your deftness would survive. Liz and Carol remember by doing for me. Bubba writes a postcard full of frantic premonition. Joe remembers saucer-blue eyes and bee-stung lips hiding a sly intelligence. Larry says you taught him to see. (Each memory's a wound.) George brings a verb. (No word can be right.) Drunk with sorrow, your Uncle Jay has called me three times (Each drink is a kiss.) . . .

Forgive, Charley, the names unnamed. (Each name is a sigh.) Even in Canada, people are telling Charley stories. How you made us smile!

I miss you,

Antonio Padial
(Tagu)

When Jerry died, my world suddenly stopped. There were no more pills to sort out, no more meals to prepare, no more sweat-soaked towels to wash, no one left to love. Only a vast, painful emptiness.

The day after he died, I made myself go to see the Quilt on display in Chicago. It was only then that I felt relief from my anger, my frustrations, my loneliness. I had a project, a way to make myself realize that it really did happen, both the good and the bad. It would be my memorial to him, my tribute to the man that I loved.

The material used was sent over from Hong Kong. Jerry and I led a rich and full existence, and the brocade was an attempt to capture that. We only had four years together, but they were packed with a lot of living and loving. We met in London while he was still living in Hong Kong. We commuted to see each other halfway across the world, and then when I finally got to Hong Kong, he was posted to Tokyo. I went on to business school in Chicago, and we still continued to see each other on average every six weeks between Tokyo and Hong Kong. We worked really hard at our relationship to make it happen, to use each stolen moment to its fullest.

When he was diagnosed with pneumonia in Tokyo, I flew with him back to Chicago for treatment. We both knew what it was and what it would mean.

He was at the peak of his career and he was simply devastated. But he was also Jerry, and his every approach to the disease was with level-headedness and stoicism. He fought it with strength, courage and dignity. After two bouts with PCP, he developed lymphoma in his lungs. Finally, his once strong body gave out about 16 months later, being continually beaten down with chemotherapy and the virus.

Jerry was usually in control. I am positive that when he knew that it was no longer worth his while to fight and continue to suffer (as did the rest of us), he just decided that enough was enough. He passed away in the middle of the night on July 10th, 1988.

Jerry will always be in the Quilt. The scenes are those that would have meant a lot to him, if he could see it. The quilt celebrates our love, his preoccupation with building himself a home to die in, my precious gift of a garden for him in his final year, and the friends who have made the burden a little easier to carry.

The message on the quilt is important to me, too. I am very tired now of crying alone. If my message of pain and love manages to touch others, then I would have succeeded and the panel would have served its purpose.

There really was a Pandabear and an Oik.

Alwyn

Ronald J. Frazier ===============

Ronald J. Frazier was born and named Andre M. in Harlem, New York, on October 26, 1948. He changed his name to protect his family from shame at the time he was given a prison sentence for a drug-related burglary in 1979. At that time he fabricated a name based on two of the black athletes that he admired most, a heavyweight champion and a basketball player.

When he entered prison he was taking a step that too many black men in our society seem to take, after a childhood of racism, poverty, an abusive stepfather, an early departure from home, at age 17, and a war experience in Vietnam. While serving time on Riker's Island, he was a witness to a murder there. For refusing to name and testify against the murderer he was charged with "acting in concert" with the killer and sentenced to life in prison. Although witnesses to his innocence later came forth, and he studied paralegal skills so that he could appeal for a new trial, his efforts to reopen his case were denied and he died of AIDS in prison.

You might ask if his life was "wasted," but the many people whose lives he touched would answer that question with a resounding NO! During his 11 years in prison he earned a college degree from SUNY, New Paltz, in 1989, just a year before he died. He planned to study social work and to work with children of families in crisis. He was a gifted artist and his drawings of people and animals were very much in demand in the prison environment.

Poetry and speechwriting were two other skills that he expressed in many different ways. He became the president of the prison student association, participated in a forum on the right to free speech in prison, and wrote a poem called "Requiem for Fallen Comrades" which the prison psychologist took to Washington and read in front of the Vietnam Veterans Memorial there, while her husband made a videotape of the event, which was later shown to a veteran's group in the prison.

One of the most difficult consequences of his early life was the loss of contact with his two daughters, which meant that he had no way of knowing how their lives were developing. He expressed his continuing love for children by participating in a fathers' group and taking parenting classes, and by spending time with other prisoners' families. One of my favorite images of him is at the end of a prison visit, when he gave a yellow rose (that I had "sneaked into the visiting room" by wearing it in my hair) to a little girl who was just parting from her father.

Ron was a spiritual seeker and we shared many letters and conversations about our connections to the universe. He loved animals and all living things and his drawings reflected this. He also formulated sharp political analyses of the larger society and of the structure within the walls of Eastern Correctional Facility. One of the last papers that he wrote before his graduation was about women's spirituality. He tutored other prisoners in literacy skills, helped with

continued

paralegal issues, and had studied and learned two languages while in prison, Spanish and American Sign Language.

I also agreed to try to be with him when he was dying and was able to spend the day and evening with him on June 5, 1990, at St. Clare's hospital prison ward. He then died, alone, on June 6, just after dawn. His sister was also able to visit him on the eve of his death but the guards denied her request to stay with him during the night, even though it was clear to all of us that he was actively dying.

It was healing for me as well as for him, to be his friend and to meet and support his mother and his sister as the time of his death from AIDS drew nearer. Our relationship also challenged my inherent racism, even though I've been doing anti-racist and civil rights work for years. It gave me a whole new perspective on the peace and justice work that is a core part of my life.

Mickie Lynn

My entire fifth grade class worked on this beautiful panel for several months. I really think that we benefited greatly from the experience. Walter Novas was a very good friend—even though we did not know him personally. Our knowledge of him came secondhand from our teacher, Mr. Clute.

AIDS is a very scary disease. Although I do not know anyone with AIDS now, it seems like I have been involved with a million people because of this quilt and because this is such a horrible virus that has killed or will kill so many. I think that everyone my age should get the education about AIDS and HIV that my class has received. We must learn the facts and work towards prevention and cure.

Beth Olson,
Room 112

September 16, 1991

JIM SMITH

I met Jim Smith in 1985 at a fledgling support group for HIV positive (then HTLV-III) individuals.

Jim was unique, an artist who had the ability to combine a free, liberal spirit with the intricacy of his work. His prize artwork was handmade detailed puppets. I believe that his art kept him going because it allowed him to escape from the virus for at least a little while.

The intensity that Jim exhibited with his art carried through into other areas of his life. We took a trip to Cancun to get isoprinosine to try and boost our immune systems. He would spend four hours at a time in the water, snorkeling, watching the tropical fish, studying the coral reefs. Since we were in a sense smuggling the drug into the U.S., we were very fearful of coming through customs. Jim was not real good at hiding his emotions. Our luggage was stuffed with isoprinosine (hundreds of dollars' worth) and we had made a pact that if one of us got through and the other got caught we still would split the stash. I'm amazed we both made it. I had never seen a person who was tan from a week in the sun look so ghostly white as he went through customs. The rush we felt when we got out of the international terminal probably did more for our immune systems than the isoprinosine! Amidst the joy, hugging and laughing, Jim had tears streaming down his face.

Jim was not a totally positive person, which is understandable, since he had debilitating problems with ARC symptoms. He was acutely in tune with his body and psyche and what changes were occurring. This is not to take away from Jim, but rather to point out that he had a keen awareness that no matter what he felt, whether positive or negative, the important thing was to allow these feelings to be expressed.

What really affected me about Jim was his deep philosophical thinking and his concern for others. When most of us were discussing what certain signs and symptoms meant to our longevity, Jim would contemplate how our lives affected the universe ("Does one life effect change? Does happiness and contentment come from within and can it be projected onto others? Is all the pain and suffering worth the struggle? . . .").

Jim showed me how to put things in perspective, probably even more so after his death when I reflect on his living. So the answer to these questions is "Yes!" We do make a difference. I miss Jim!

David G. Brey

P.S.: The significance of the raccoon on the panel is that Jim had a stuffed toy raccoon at his bedside whenever he was hospitalized.

Nowadays, the back of the weekly publication "This Week in Texas" has at least a page or two of obituaries. In spite of the fear and dread I feel each time I pick one up, I always look there first to see if anyone I know is listed. It was a nasty shock to find my friend Isaias "Ike" Rodriguez, Jr. smiling at me from his obituary.

Because of demands on my time as panel-making coordinator for the San Antonio Chapter of the NAMES Project, I returned to the workshop one evening after it was closed to work in private on Ike's panel.

As a finishing touch, I decided to outline Ike's name with this shiny black paint that has to be squeezed out of the nozzle of a little plastic bottle. I worked my way down one side and was most of the way back up the other side, too engrossed in the trees to see the forest, when I noticed the black smudges on my arm. Of course, they were on the panel as well, and my heart just sank and my stomach just churned. My first impulse was simply to say "the hell with it" and start all over again. It didn't do much good trying to cover the smudges with a red marker.

Then I thought about my friend Ike. We enrolled in cosmetology school together, went through all our 1,500 hours and sometimes even rode to and from school together. Ike simply was not the sort of person to take any extra pains to get something done. Every time he was assigned to do a shampoo and roller set, he managed to talk his client into letting him use a blowdryer and curling iron instead. The more I thought about it, the better I remembered the extent to which he served as a counterpoint to my fastidiousness and how bemused he always was at my exasperation over his ways. There were different ways Ike could routinely be sloppy about certain things (except his own hair!). He was just a lot more interested in going about his way of having a good time and enjoying life than in anything else. And if he burned his candle at both ends, it *did*, as the poem says, make a lovely light.

That was when I decided to leave the panel just as it was, black smears and all. After all, it's *Ike's* panel—why should it be perfect? I think Ike's chin *was* there on my shoulder, prodding my arm into the wet paint to remind me that life is too short to take things so seriously.

The stark color contrast in the panel represents his hot, impulsive Aries nature interacting with my own cool, rational Libran self. We had some hot, unforgettable times!

Rafael L. Jimenez

Dear John, Here I sit in China's World, slaving over my morning cup of coffee. Sure do miss you, buddy . . .

Well, John, you know how I dread putting pen to paper. It's so much easier to pick up the phone. Sure wish I could this time. I think I'll start closing here, before I get mushy on you. Anyway, you already knew of the love, friendship and understanding we both had between us. Your life they couldn't save, but the memories are forever.

Take care, sweetie, wherever you are, till we meet again.

Love always,
Donuts
(Debbie Canfield)

September 11, 1987

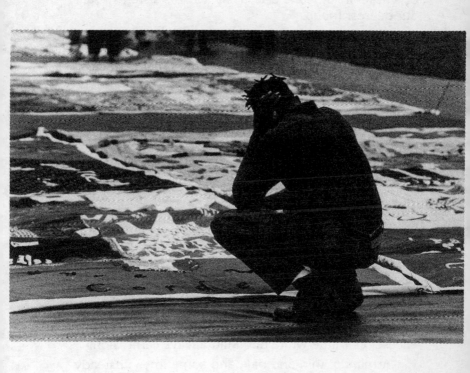

Armando Cotayo was our friend. We knew him as you know people who live in other cities but are close by virtue of someone else. That was his sister, Rosa, our dearest friend.

Eight months before his death, we all took a trip together, to the beach. In the face of sickness and increasing frailty, Armando displayed great courage. Slowly shaping the interior life that the dying build for themselves, Armando still reached out to make his friends feel welcome.

A group of us drove from Tucson to Puerto Penasco, through dry desert to a pristine stretch of shoreline just inside the Mexican border. Privately we all wished that a sunny and boisterous weekend would be a kind of forgetting.

Every morning, we woke to cool breezes. The sky was endless and seemed to stretch across the top half of the earth and the ocean outside our door shone like a field of wet turquoise. After coffee and rolls and minute discussions about tan lines and body lotions, we would wander down to the beach and unpack umbrellas, blankets, frisbees, cold soda, lotion, hats, fishing poles, potato chips, oranges, magazines, beer, cheese. Our little white dog Miki always came along.

Armando, thin and pale and sometimes unsteady on his feet, set a jaunty straw hat on his head and slowly padded to the beach with the rest of us. He read, laughed and watched the swimmers pedal away from shore. In the afternoon he slept and at night he ate dinner with the noisy group and talked about work, though he was not working by then; food, though he was rarely hungry; movies he might never see.

One night, late, after a dinner of grilled "blue" shrimp, frijoles and beer, Rosa drifted onto the terrace. The sky was filled with stars. She wept. And it was Armando who shuffled outside and put his arms around her. He consoled her. He embraced her. He teased her. He told her it would be OK. And we imagined, that night, the two of them as kids: Armando, the big brother, telling his little sister in the middle of an urgent adolescent crisis that everything would be OK. They probably spoke in Spanish. They probably talked fast, finishing each other's sentences, and they almost certainly teased each other.

It was a lovely sight, that night, in Puerto Penasco. Arms locked, tears dry, Armando and Rosa faced the ocean, looking up into the black sky, speaking Spanish, talking fast, laughing. It was a fine moment to remember.

Jacqi Tully,
Nadia Ruimy,
Linda Kropowensky

James was born and raised in Akron, Ohio. He was a good-looking black man about 5′7″ tall. He was from a very poor and uneducated family. James had a very tough childhood and lived part of his life in foster homes. When he was old enough he joined the Army and was stationed in Germany.

He met a young woman there and fell in love. He told me that was the only woman he ever loved. The Army refused to give them permission to get married because she had a police record and a history of drug use. By that time, James had gotten into the drug scene himself. He returned to the U.S. and worked many low-paying jobs. He never really got out of the rut where his life began.

I met James after I received a call and was asked to go visit a young man who had contracted the HIV virus from using IV drugs. James was still able to get around pretty well but the conditions he was living under were horrible. The house was filthy and there were usually just a couple of kids there when I went to see him. One day he called me and asked me to come over right away. By this time he had become bedfast.

When I got there flies were all over him because he had an accident and no one would clean him up. There was no hot water so I carried him to the car and brought him to my home, gave him a bath and put clean clothes on him.

I only knew James for about three months. I would have never gotten to know him had he not become sick. I became his friend and grew to like him a lot. I remember one day he reached over and grabbed my hand and said, "You're alright." It made me feel so good to know I had been there for him. It never bothered him that I was gay. He was a product of poverty who was never able to get out of the ghetto he was born in. He helped me realize there is good in all of us, that even a drug addict is a worthwhile human being in need of a helping hand.

James told me one evening he was ready to go, that he was tired of struggling. The next time I saw him he wasn't able to respond, he just stared at the ceiling. He died the next day [age 29].

Rev. Karl Selman

April 20, 1978. That was the day I first started with the phone company. I was to be an operator. Jimmy sat down next to me. We talked for a bit and I knew right away that I had found a friend. It was nice to have someone to talk to and share a giggle with. Being new in town, I had really missed having someone that I could play and be silly with. Jimmy gave me that.

Jackie Kennedy was his idol. On a costume day at work, he finally got an opportunity to wear his pink pillbox hat and little white gloves.

I talked to Jimmy only a few days before he died. I was glad to have the opportunity to tell him how much I loved him. His mother said his face was covered in tears so I know that he was able to understand what I said. By that time he could not speak, only nod and cry.

I am glad to have had Jimmy in my life. I miss him. So many times I look at his picture and I have to laugh. Jimmy would have been laughing with me.

Love,
Anna Damiani

Please accept my panel in memory of my lover John Fay. I realize that the panel does not fit the designated 3′ × 6′. As in our lives and relationship he refused to be bound by conventions, so in death I must let others supply the definition, make the measure and take according to their needs.

I doubt I'll ever find another so thoughtful, loving and giving. I wish I could send a photo—of course there are none. John was always the one behind the camera, creating the situation, recording the scene, striving to illuminate the nuances passed over by others. I wish I had occasionally overridden his protestations and captured his likeness, either composed or spontaneous or surreptitious. Even in my mind's eye I see him most recently and sick, and it's hard to remember back even a few years to another time—does one ever *REALLY* look? It's hard to remember.

This is very difficult.

Brian O'Regan

October 9, 1987

PAUL GIANNOBILE, JR. ══════════

When he was with us, Paul Giannobile, Jr. was: Son, brother, friend, lover, movie fan/critic, fashion plate, decorator, accessorizer, collector, dancer, party giver, partygoer, biker, sunbather, cook, waiter, host, music lover, traveller, bon vivant, trendsetter/spotter.

He was a "first-sight soul-shaking, one-night lovemaking, next-day heartbreaking guy." Now that he's left us he's much more.

Robert Huckaby

Our local AIDS support group (Polk AIDS Support Services) received a phone call that a young man in jail was being released from jail because he had AIDS. We were asked to try to locate housing for him, which we attempted to do. His condition worsened, and he was transferred to the County Hospital, where he immediately died.

We never met Clarence. We never even got to talk to him. He was gone so quickly. We know nothing about Clarence.

His quilt is in memory of a man who otherwise would not have been remembered in the AIDS epidemic.

Webster Benner, Jr.
and Harriet Benner

Ronald Earl Mitchell checked into this penal colony planet Midsummers Eve at high noon July 31, 1950. It cost $50 at Tampa General Hospital, Tampa, Florida.

Checked out at 7:50 p.m., April 4, 1985, from M.D. Anderson Hospital, at the phenomenal cost of $52,734.

The usual bratty child graduated Galena Park Tex High School joining the Coast Guard. Two years later he came home with a squawking parrot on his shoulder and an earring in his ear.

For the remainder of his life he joined the Frame Factory chain and also U-Frame-It and became a master picture framer.

He was a gentle brown-eyed man. 5'8"; very muscular.

A tender, caring person who never hurt a living thing. He had a green thumb and loved gardening.

He loved birds. Had a large pink cockatoo, plenty of cockatiels and finches. He was psychic . . . studying the occult and the Tarot. Twice he saved my life with his pre-vision.

He was creative. He could take any old piece of junk and turn it into a thing of beauty. He was a dancing fool, and loved to disco. Astoundingly enough, he loved to take his mother along (as flashy as possible).

continued

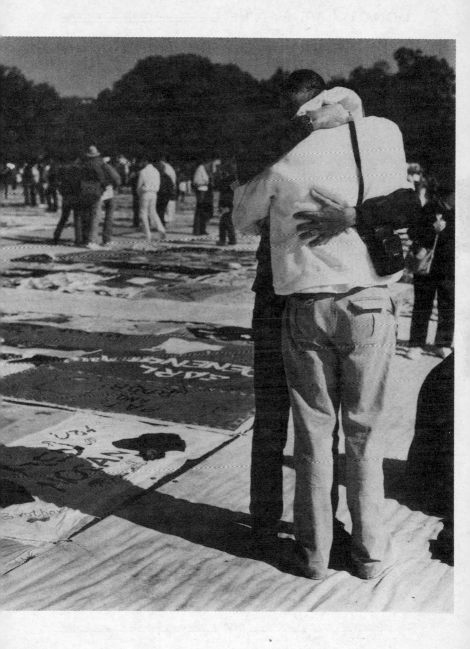

He lived life intensely because he knew it would be short. He was exciting to be around. In short, he was a beautiful spirit . . . alive or dead.

I'm sorry God needed him for a tour of duty somewhere else!!

His loving mother,
Yolanda Y. Mitchell

P.S.: His panel, done but poorly by me, is his own work. I merely traced, enlarged and transferred it to his panel.

It is a dream he had often. He etched it and framed it in stained glass. It hangs in my picture window as my most prized possession.

His panel is his tombstone and only immortality . . . he has no grave.

His picture and his ashes rest on his piano at my side. That way I may put flowers and keep a candle burning brightly as my love for him as long as I survive.

He was no Rock Hudson or Liberace, but he *was* talented. Who knows how that might have grown in the years that were taken from him?

It seems to me that the light of the whole world is slowly dying with this monstrous plague—destroying millions of our greatest talents with it. Can it be one of the great plagues prophesied in Revelations?

We can only wonder.

I went to school with Dan at the Atlanta College of Art. He was a painter, and, like me, a procrastinator.

I liked him—and I identified with him. We both took more than four years to graduate—he was so happy on his graduation day. Dan was 30 years old when he died last year of AIDS-related meningitis. I heard someone say after his death that he hadn't accomplished much—I didn't know him well, but I always found him to be kind, good-humored and very creative—I think that is enough.

My life partner and I had to stay up the night before the march to finish his panel—I think he would have thought that was funny—he would have done the same thing.

Karen Chance

I miss my brother, Kenneth. It has been three years, almost to the day, since he died and there remains a profound sadness to my life without him.

Oh, he wasn't around much. His life was filled with activity and people—much the way mine is, I suppose. In fact, he seemed to draw activity and people—a base, a touchstone of sorts, to those around him. But he was always there when it counted. Those times when we came together as family—when our individual orbits were purposely synchronized for togetherness on birthdays and holidays. I miss him most then—his laughing eyes and often wry grin; the tender, true way he was able to interact with my children, who also still mourn his loss.

My youngest daughter was not quite three when Kenneth died. I thought she was too young to understand or be hurt by the experience. Yet she still cries at night occasionally, and it is a special sound she makes. I always know it is about Kenneth and not a tummyache or one of life's other injustices. He touched her as he seemed to touch nearly everyone he knew, and she knows that she lost something precious when he died.

Kenneth was vibrant and dynamic; someone who could make things happen when the world around him was steeped in inertia. He had a gift for life. It was heart-wrenching to watch him die.

He was so many things you should know about. He was creative and charming, sensitive and thoughtful. He was selfish in his own way and I'm glad. Because he was able to take so much more from life in 26 years than most of us will in a lifetime. For my oldest daughter's fourth birthday he brought balloons, hundreds of the big, expensive balloons in rich, sassy colors of the rainbow. And a tank of helium. It was a splendid day of color, filled with perfect photographs of fun. It was like Kenneth: bright and memorable, with more than a touch of whimsy. But, as was his custom, he left before the party had ended—in pursuit, no doubt, of his next adventure . . .

Linda Fermoyle Rice

At the center of each display of the Quilt is the signature square, a 12' × 12' expanse of blank fabric, where visitors to the quilt are invited to kneel on the square and leave their own memorial, message or mark.

From signature squares around the country:

. . . I don't think I knew what I was in for or what I would see. I felt like a fool crying but at the end I figured out that it was expected.

E.

What an honor to be in the presence of so much love.

Jennifer

They say that if only one person is touched by seeing this Quilt, then it has accomplished its purpose. But the truth is that we are all touched. Today is the day the ignorance dies and the compassion begins.

Jeremiah

I found tears in my eyes and a lump in my throat. These were real people—they will never ever be just names or numbers to me anymore. They were husbands, fathers, brothers, and friends, and so much more. This experience reminds me of the Vietnam memorial, except this is so much more personal and special . . . I will pray for these victims and their families tonight, as well as for some of my friends who I fear may be at risk . . .

Goodbye, Uncle Tom. I love you.

Kim

The Quilt brings the people to life. It's about time society realizes it's not just statistics. Thank you for the realization.

Chris

Any one of you could have been any one of my friends. I won't forget.

Mollie

I thought I would learn to better accept death but instead I found a passion for life. Do not let dreams die.

Mindy

Mickey,
You are always in my heart—someday we'll be together again. I love you so much.
Your sister,

Carole

I don't know many. I hope to know only a few more. I wish there weren't any to know.

Dan

I have always been almost repulsed by AIDS and the people who carry it. I now embrace these people, and the disease. I see now that these people are the same as you and me! I have been deeply moved by this experience! Keep the faith!

Sandi

May this Quilt extinguish the shadow of ignorance and fear that paralyzes so many. The Quilt lights a lamp of hope. May it shine until the deaths are no more.

R.H.

It's terribly difficult to deal with the flood of emotions from these sections of memory. The love meets the pain head-on and tears seem to be the only adequate symbols.

Scott

Why is it only that in death we can see the value of life. I feel as if I knew you all.

A.M.P.

I read until the tears blurred the words. Then, I just felt. I love you all, my new friends.

Mathew

From their death comes beauty
From their memory comes hope
You have opened my eyes and broken
my heart

Betty C.

I pray that my children never see and
cry over this Quilt. May there be a solution
soon.

Jodie

I am numb with fear. Once my
numbness subsides, I will be driven to act.

Sally

We understand!

Jenny and Katie

My Own Little Message

From December 1 (World AIDS Day) through December 9, 1990, a portion of the AIDS Memorial Quilt was on display in the Capital District of New York State for the first time—in the Terrace Gallery, fourth floor, at the New York State Museum.

In early November, I decided to be a volunteer at the Quilt exhibit, even though I had not, at that time, ever seen the Quilt except via videotape of the Inaugural Display of the Quilt in Washington, D.C., on October 11, 1987. Though the medium of TV is certainly nothing like being there, I saw for the first time hints of what the Quilt means and how its viewers and creators responded to it.

I attended a one-hour training session with dozens of other prospective volunteers in a large white meeting room at the Museum on November 18. After the information session, where the presenter passed out literature and answered questions, some of us walked slowly and quietly to part of the meeting room where one section of eight 3′ × 6′ panels, sewed into a 12′ × 12′ square, lay unfolded on the floor.

I felt some sadness as I gazed at that square, my first-ever glimpse of part of the Quilt. It looked so lonely there, with no other sections around it. In the brightly lit meeting room, the colors of the eight panels stood out and seemed to impress everyone who gazed at them. After a time, I ambled away from the square, feeling reverent and having the odd sensation of "abandoning" it. Still, it provided help in preparing me emotionally for my first viewing of hundreds of panels of the Quilt.

continued

My Own Little Message

On Friday, November 30 at 5 p.m., the AIDS Memorial Quilt exhibit "opened" . . . As soon as I got off the elevator, I could already see dozens of panels of the Quilt—some were on the floor, but most were suspended with thin cables from the high ceiling. Immediately, I was awed by the variety of colors, materials, styles, and details of the panels . . .

As I stood near one particular panel (about three feet away—a respectful distance, I hoped), I began to feel an emptiness, a sadness. The panel spelled out a victim's name on a simulated Scrabble board, complete with word and letter-score squares and numeric point values for the letters of the person's name. I am a Scrabble player, and felt sad that this unknown (to me) person who died at probably a young age and probably with much pain and suffering, would never be able to play Scrabble with me—or do anything—with anyone, again. The panel, like virtually all I saw, was very colorful and meticulously crafted, but it lay very still, very flat against the partition. I could feel tears in my eyes, feel them start to slide down my face as I slowly wandered among the panels, thinking of the grieving, the loving, the caring persons who made certain that their loved ones, close friends, and family members would be remembered in the nicest, most dignified, most moving—and imaginative—ways that could be expressed in 18 square feet of fabric. . . . I tried to "see" and "hear" the persons commemorated in the panels, tried to imagine what their lives were like, what they could or would say if they could have been viewing the Quilt as

I was. Perhaps, somehow, they are—and we just don't know how or from where . . .

I found much more cheer than if I were at a cemetery, viewing these same names and short lives of persons who died of AIDS. Instead of the flowing and beautifully blended variety of colors, there would only be stark grays, tans, whites. Instead of fabric and other materials associated with warmth and color, there would only be hard, cold tombstones and monuments. Instead of the names of places and objects that were cherished by the deceased, and sometimes the inclusion of actual objects such as teddy bears, clothes, and photographs, a cemetery would contain only names and dates, no mention of what the lives of the deceased were like, where they traveled, what they enjoyed . . . One would have to travel to a cemetery—perhaps hundreds or thousands of miles—to view those names. Instead of being surrounded by many caring, fellow viewers of the Quilt and volunteers who would give hugs and lend support to viewers, a cemetery would likely be deserted, a place of acute silence and loneliness, with only a very few or one living soul among the deceased . . .

In a corner of the Gallery, an isolated square of the Quilt had hundreds of messages written all over its 12′ × 12′ expanse, with "The NAMES Project" in very large block lettering over much of the square. Gently, I knelt by one edge of the square, and slowly and carefully penned in my own little message, using a blue marking pen:

continued

"Mario, I am sad that AIDS never gave you a chance for us to share good times and memories. Love and missing you, John."

I bowed my head and stared at the sad little message to my former colleague for several minutes. I did not cry or whimper, I just remained still and numb. Then I stood slowly, and as I did so, many more little messages of remembrance came into my field of vision, slightly blurred by welling tears. I read some of the other messages, then walked past the remainder of the Quilt, solemnly gazing at the representation of what is probably the worst peacetime tragedy in our country in decades, the AIDS epidemic . . .

On a wall opposite the exit door, I gazed at the newest panels of the Quilt. Sad that there have to be any, and sad that there are AIDS victims without panels to commemorate them. Lack of money. Lack of faith, or courage, or resources or even desire by those who loved or knew them. Most panels have one or two names. One of the latest panels contained dozens of names, strung together in script style. Mostly first names. Even in death, some persons remain anonymous for a variety of reasons . . .

On Sunday evening, I attended a "Celebration of Life" benefit in the lobby level of the museum. I was very pleased that over 400 people attended this fundraising event for agencies involved in the fight against AIDS and trying to make the lives of people living with AIDS more bearable and comfortable. There was a private viewing of the Quilt, so I again viewed it for a while, then rejoined the party in the lobby three floors below. For indeed, it feels good to celebrate life, to be alive, to help persons in need of it, and to help fund the effort to eradicate AIDS somehow, someday.

Then, no more panels will be added to the Quilt. I hope that as many people as possible will see the *last* panel added, for that will be a powerful symbol of the time when AIDS is finally conquered, the time that no more people—men and women, young and old, gay, straight, bisexual—die of AIDS, its complications, or its opportunistic infections.

In the meantime, there is the Quilt. May its message and meaning become known to all humankind.

John W. Morse

December 6, 1990

CHARLES C. KOEHLER, JR. ══════════

Chuck Koehler was one of four children. He is survived by two brothers, Paul and Allen, and a sister, Norah.

Chuck always knew what he wanted to do, and followed through, beginning with grammar, high school, and college. He served three-and-one-half years as a Navy corpsman and has an honorable discharge from the Vietnam War era.

Chuck loved the good life, and with his lover, Jim, maintained the best life of home, travel, and friends. Jim died of AIDS eight months before Chuck was taken by the same much-dreaded AIDS.

My son was always there for me and anyone who needed him. He had a beautiful sense of humor, a compassionate soul, and an extremely wonderful mind. He would kid me (his mom) all the time about my cooking, my thrifty shopping habits. Paper towels, cheese, and crackers were not on his list. He liked the best—fine wines, good cuts of meat, and chocolate desserts.

Chuck could win anyone so easy as a friend. He would talk your ear off about any issue and never make you feel small. His smile, soft voice, and clear eyes told everyone he was a nice man to know.

He never lied about his lifestyle, he was proud and content to be gay. He always said he would not die of embarrassment and he did not. He freely told everyone from his work to friends when he became HIV-positive and then came down with AIDS.

Chuck planned his life and did all he planned right up to the week before he died. He even tried to tell Rev. Hamilton of St. Paul's United Methodist, how to do the service for him.

Chuck will walk gently through our hearts for a long time as he touched so many and is still touching people, like his Mothers of AIDS Patients group, special friends at St. Paul's United Methodist, and Being Alive support group. He left so many close friends, he was truly rich with their love.

Chuck will be desperately missed by his mom, who had more quiet moments holding hands and talking about each other's special thoughts. I'm one mom who can truly say, "Chuck and I had it all," but not long enough.

Mom
(Kathryn B. Koehler)

Michael Crowley was my brother. We were 16 months apart. We were so close growing up that people used to ask us if we ever fought . . .

He meant . . . means . . . more to me than I can express on this paper. He taught me . . . how to write, how to understand, how to appreciate . . . and mostly he taught me how to think. He educated those around him gently, tactfully, with humor. He saw deeper; he knew when you were hurting . . .

He was a survivor of a difficult young life. He attended Williams College and brought home much more than a degree. He gave our family pride.

When he graduated he went across the country with his best friend—he stretched his mind, he pushed himself forward. He worked as a mental health worker, and then he decided on law school. He became a lawyer in 1986 . . . he found out he was sick eight months before graduation. He graduated with his lover watching in the audience . . . his lover died seven months later. He knew complete joy and complete heartbreak.

When he got sick none of us believed it could ever really happen. We couldn't trust our own instincts. We were sure he wouldn't get so sick that death would even become a possibility. He died October 21, 1987.

I can't write any more about him because it is becoming too hard to share him. I love him very much. I always told him I was "him" in female form.

My grief is too great to bear sometimes, but he would love to know his panel would be part of the project. He worked on one for his lover six months before he died. He saw a picture of it in Washington three days before he died.

The joy he gave me will be a difficult gift to repay. I feel I owe him something. I would do anything for him. And now the only thing I can do is to carry on his cause . . . help people to understand and tell them we all have to work very hard so that other "sisters" like me don't have to feel the sadness I feel . . .

Laurie Ann Leone

Oh, Lord! The images and memories of 20 years flood out welcome and unwanted at the same time.

Jim loved circuses, Christmas, Jon, J.D., tacky things, Sondheim shows, Barbara Cook and Timi Yuro, a little Wagner and a lot of Janis Joplin. Jim was our first friend to die, back in the days when we all thought AIDS was an FBI/CIA plot to quarantine and exterminate us.

Jim could be difficult at times, a joy at others. Sometimes a drag, but always busy and on the go. Just like us all.

Why can't I say more about our best friend? I don't know. It's still painful, and I am hurt and angry.

This panel helps.

Bryon Predika

Sarah Anne Schmitz was born in Waukegan, Illinois, on January 18, 1987. I don't think I need to tell you what a precious gift she was to me. Sarah was happy and smiling most of the time.

Sarah was "officially" diagnosed with AIDS-related complex at eight months old.

Sarah was the most incredible little girl! She was very beautiful. She had a profound effect on everybody with whom she came in contact. We thought she was special, of course, but at her funeral, people from every part of her life were in attendance.

Sarah didn't live very long, but she accomplished some incredible things. She taught us about acceptance, living "one day at a time" and UNCONDITIONAL LOVE. She was extremely patient with her parents as they learned what parenting was all about.

Sarah loved Sesame Street. Big Bird was her favorite. She liked Cubs baseball. She loved bright colors and pretty things. She liked makeup and jewelry. She loved her doggie Lisa and her kitty Rufus.

She stayed with us until she "just couldn't love anymore." She was too tired. She lived and died at home. She died a peaceful death in Mommy's arms. Daddy was there, too.

We love you, Sarah,

Julianne Schmitz

Enclosed with this letter is a quilt panel for my lover, Rusty Vega.

His full name is Milton Edgardo Vega Garcia Serrano Quinones Figueroa Soto Mayor, but because of his beautiful auburn hair and freckles, we call him Rusty.

Born September 21, 1960, in Adjuntas, Puerto Rico, his family moved to New York when Rusty was six years old. He lived there in the Bronx and Manhattan until he was 21 and met me. I swept him off to Los Angeles for three years, and then San Francisco for five. This is where he died.

In New York, he was primarily a waiter in some of the city's finest restaurants, among them Claire, Joanna's, and J.G. Melons in Bridgehampton. In L.A., he worked at En Brochette, Neimann-Marcus, and Robinson's Beverly Hills. One of his proudest positions was working for the Organizing Committee for the 1984 Olympic Games, where attending opening ceremonies was the fulfillment of a lifelong dream. In San Francisco, he was a merchandise planner for The Gap, Inc., a position he held until his illness disabled him in March 1989.

Rusty and my relationship can be defined as love at first sight for both of us. Within two weeks of meeting each other in New York, we were living together in Los Angeles. For both of us, it was the premier relationship of either of our lives. We were desperately in love from the moment we met until he died in my arms on the morning of November 30, 1989, a period of about seven and a half years.

This quilt panel was designed by myself and Russ Butler, an artist and friend of us both, and was sewn by Jutta Linn in Laguna Beach. We made it to represent Rusty into history and our love for him into eternity. He'll never die for me, in my heart and in my memory, and now he'll never be forgotten as a result of his being immortalized in the Quilt.

Thanks,

Sam Coco

For Rusty
Back again to your City by the Bay,
Where usually I come to play
And climb your hills and touch your sky,
But this time I come to say goodbye.

Farewell to a friend that I knew well,
About whose friendship I come to tell.
He loved his life from day to day;
We used to dance the nights away.
He made friendship into an art,
This little man with a giant heart.

continued

Someone to accept me—right or wrong
Or tell me that my hair's too long,
Or what I should or shouldn't wear;
It's nice to know that he was there.
I wore his clothes, which he'd allow—
I'm even wearing his shirt right now.
Through those of us he leaves behind
He'll live forever in our mind.

Oh, God, please let this sad song end
Before we lose another friend.
Please cause the dreaded plague to cease
That all may live full lives in peace
With strength and hope and dignity,
Not having to think—that this could be me—
Or fade away in secrecy.

So I'm back to the City by the Sea
Though it's just not quite the same to me.
The hills are still here, as is each tree,
And life still holds on desperately.
Yet high above the gull and the dove
This well-remembered soul flies free.

Your friend,

Russell "the King" Butler

After being asked to do an issues project on the topic of discrimination, we chose to examine the topic of AIDS. We felt as though AIDS patients often experience unnecessary discrimination and their needs and feelings are often overlooked. All of us wanted to reach out to try to understand those who have and will fall victim to this disease as well as to show others to do the same.

After viewing the film "Common Threads," we were deeply moved and decided to make a quilt patch in honor of the five children in Massachusetts who have died of AIDS. This would be a form of reaching out to the many family members of AIDS victims and showing them how much we supported and felt for them. AIDS, a disease unmercifully preying on the human race, has reached home in numerous places around the world. Deaths of many are closer to home than we may think. Massachusetts, the state in which we live, is full of innocent people whose lives have been taken.

Our quilt patch stands as a reminder to people of all ages that AIDS is a very serious problem that won't just go away. We, as a community, have to decide what we can do to help people with AIDS and what we can do to prevent the spread of the disease. Knowing that others are concerned with their welfare might encourage people to protect themselves and their offspring from AIDS. Drug users, people engaging in sexual relations, doctors, everyone should be aware of the rapid spread of AIDS, and to be concerned not only for themselves but for each other.

Students at
Milton Academy
Middle School

REINO MARTTILA, JR. ========

The enclosed quilt panel was made in honor of Reino (Ray-no) Marttila, Jr. Had Reino not been a person with AIDS, I may never have met him. As a volunteer in the Buddy Program of the San Diego AIDS Project, I was assigned to Reino soon after I completed my volunteer training in July of 1985.

Over the nearly 14 months that we had together, we grew very close, even interdependent, our moods affecting each other. He listened to my joys and sorrows as much as I listened to his, and those times that we shared are among the most valued that I've ever had. Whether we went out to lunch, to the doctor's office, shopping, or just stayed home and cuddled on the couch, I came away feeling uplifted.

I entered the relationship expecting to be the nurturer, the giver. But Reino was also a skilled giver. No matter how sick he was, he found the words to touch my heart. Little statements such as "I'm so glad you're here," or, "You always make things better" fixed up my whole day.

Once when he was particularly ill, I lay down beside him on his bed and held his frail body close to mine until he stopped shivering. He said, "Oh, God, I didn't think anyone would ever hold me again." His words made me realize the enormity of the isolation he had endured since his diagnosis. I knew that if I tried to speak, I would cry. We did a lot more holding after that.

Reino's final weeks were spent in a hospital,

gradually succumbing to pneumonia. During that period we spent many silent hours just holding hands, no longer needing to speak. From time to time he would awaken with a start, and ask if someone else was standing at his bedside. Once he pointed to a solid wall and asked if there was a door there. I knew that he was very close to his transition and was trying to let me know.

I spent his final night with him, listening to the pattern of his labored breathing, and hoping each time that it faltered that it would not begin again. At six a.m., though he was still in a coma, I took him into my arms and said, "I know that it is time for you to rest now. We'll miss you very much. We'll cry and grieve and support one another. But it's OK for you to go." In less than an hour he had made his transition.

I was deeply honored that Reino allowed me to be part of this most intimate experience of letting go. He was not an educated man, but he taught me much. He was materially poor, but he found something to give. Now that I, too, am a person with AIDS, I am more fully aware of how he has prepared me. I know that he will assist me in my transition . . .

Thank you for the healing work that you are doing and for providing a vehicle through which I can express my grief.

Love in the struggle,

Robert "Jess" Jessop

February 12, 1988

There are a few really original people born into this world. David was one of these. His special combination of professional ability, energy, and a quality of living life with an intensity given only to a few made him a rare original.

David gave off a kind of buoyant energy, laughed a lot at his own foibles, but there was also a deep side that seemed uncertain of the very things he carried off so easily in the eyes of others.

This contradiction, a kind of tragic comedian, is perhaps a fair analysis of his special living style. His energy was such a part of his professional achievements. His own design firm did accomplish some large projects. His living space was ample, tasteful, and ambitious. His collections were colorful and well-chosen. Truly, he had so much to live for.

David maintained a brand of youth that would tire and baffle the youthful. His singing, his creativity, his risk-taking are legendary to all of us who entered his life . . .

As Pat Schildknecht, David's longtime friend, wrote and spoke in a eulogy:

We're going to miss this sparkplug, this guru of fun, this light in our lives, this truly eccentric, marvelous friend. Knowing David has been quite an experience.

Losing him is almost unbearable.
Forgetting him will be impossible.
We are all blessed to have had such a precious love.

Paul F. Samuelson

"Tall, dark and handsome—a little *short*, but tall, dark and handsome," said the man brushing by in a teeming bar one night. He *was* short, but hearing that put Lewayne on top of the world.

Lewayne *liked* feeling on top of the world. And when he did, he couldn't keep it to himself; he lit up like a Christmas tree on antidepressants. But he didn't often feel that way—being black and gay gave him pride and pain in equal intense measure.

He had style without pretense, a sunny sense of humor and a fierce determination to get all that was coming to him. He wanted most of all to be loved—and he was—but he never felt it . . .

Love was one of the things Lewayne could dish out but found hard to take—especially if it wasn't perfect (and when is it ever perfect?).

The full name on his birth certificate (I saw it and it's true) was Startling Lewayne Matthews, but he had grown up thinking his first name was Starling. A starling is a small dark gregarious bird with iridescent plumage and startling means surprising or dramatic. Either way, it works.

He first got sick right after he left me in 1983. (We had lived together almost since the day we met, four and a half years earlier. We had problems, but lack of love wasn't one of them.) At that same time, even though he had never performed, he eagerly joined a small troupe assembled to develop and present a stage version of an Oscar Wilde poem. The enthusiasm he carried with him set the tone for the whole project. His mysterious illness forced him to miss a couple of

continued

shows, but he just *had* to play the final performance.
"The show must go on" and, besides, his ex-lover
would be there.

Two and a half years after that, finally diagnosed
with AIDS and frightfully sick, Lewayne and I were
back together for the second time since the breakup.
Now it was time to suspend his chemotherapy and
have a nurse assigned for frequent visits.

One Sunday evening between Christmas and his
37th and last birthday, a dozen friends crowded into
his mini-studio apartment. We were certainly an oddly
cast group, reflecting the wide range of Lewayne's
affections. WE would never have chosen to be
together—what we had in common was Lewayne.

Lewayne was by then too weak, was wasting too
fast, to be left alone, but he wanted to remain at
home. So we posted a "duty roster" on the
refrigerator—and there was not an empty "shift" until
he died.

For those two months Lewayne's devoted cadre
made certain our buddy spent no night and ate no
meal alone, unless Lewayne wanted it that way. (He
never did, but then he'd never have told us if he did.)
Night after night, one of us sacked out in a sleeping
bag so when he woke to go to the bathroom, someone
he trusted would be there to help.

For me, the worst came when the virus began to
whittle away at his brain. He had always been quick,
and was proud of it, but now he was calling a drinking
straw—he could no longer hold a glass—a "salon."
Neither virus nor cancer ever darkened his smile,

though. That is, until one day when he just *stopped* smiling. The next day he stopped breathing. Maybe they were the same thing to him.

We all learned a lot in those few months—about sickroom procedures, about AIDS, about resources, about each other, about ourselves, about dying and death, about pride and courage and strength. Characteristically, Lewayne was chagrined at the "inconvenience" he was causing, but none of us could have chosen to be anywhere else . . . The "inconvenience" ended when Lewayne died.

He wouldn't even let us have a memorial but he couldn't stop us from having a party. Everyone there knew we would not meet again as a group. Most of the bond between us had died with Lewayne, but the trust and respect remained—along with pride in what we had felt and been through together. And the love we shared for our friend Lewayne.

Since that time—it's been 18 months—I've been on a voyage of discovery and rediscovery, charting the rough seas of grief with the compass of my own journal and the *startling* one Lewayne left behind. It's a hard expedition—full of unexpected monsters, typhoons, whirlpools—but I wouldn't think of turning back. Anything I can learn about Lewayne, even if it's hard to take, is worth the most arduous voyage. Besides, if I had wanted smooth sailing, I'd have chosen to love someone ordinary.

Nothing about Lewayne was ordinary.

Vincent Cage

I didn't know David for a very long time, although I'm sure I would have if given the chance. He was only 22 years old and obviously quite ill when I met him. He walked with a cane—the result of taking an experimental drug for AIDS. He came up and talked to me when I showed up at a benefit in Oakland and didn't know anyone there. That's the kind of person he was. When we went to see a play about people with AIDS at the Zephyr Theatre in San Francisco, *he* was comforting *me*! That's the kind of person he was. A kinder, more considerate person than the machos who referred to him as "faggot." A better, more deserving person than the ignorant who felt that he "asked for it" because of his lifestyle.

Joyce Biernat and I were the last people to see him alive, two hours before he died. We talked to him and hope that on some level he heard us speaking to him.

All I can say now is: What a complete and total waste!

Janet Roche,
a friend

Dear NAMES Project,

The enclosed quilt panel was made by me for my dearest friend and lover Lawrence Lott. Larry lived in Los Angeles and died at his parents' home in Greeley, Colorado, on January 24, 1991. He was 40 years old. It's quite comforting to know that a piece of him will live forever in the Quilt.

Thank you so for being there. I know you understand my grief and love.

In union with all who live during this epidemic and with all who've died,

Ana Dittmar

Tom was my spouse. We lived together five years. In that all too short time we loved, fought, built a real estate business, had an old English sheepdog, bought a house and cottage, planted fruit trees, traveled extensively in Mexico. He was my life and my happiness . . .

Matchmaking was a hobby. He wanted everyone to have someone to love and come home to in the evenings. He didn't want anyone to be alone.

I nursed him throughout his illness. His parents came to live with us for the last three months. It wasn't always easy . . .

Tom never talked about his suffering or death . . . his concerns always seemed to revolve around me. He was the most selfless and giving man I have ever met and I will always love him. He is the love of my life and I thank God I was able to have him in my life . . . he will be with me always.

William R. Reichmann

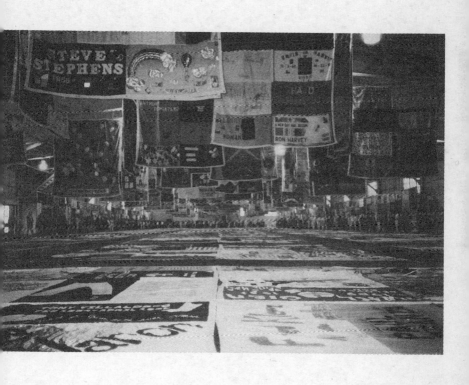

This panel for Ron Ross is the work of love from the Dayton NAMES Project's first workshop. Ronnie was a very private, but fun person who never asked for help and had to be assisted anonymously by friends.

The uniqueness of his panel is that it was made by a PWA from his support group who is also quiet and private and spent a day by himself creating this tribute to Ronnie all by himself, afraid that Ronnie would be forgotten. This panel was made by Steve Shores.

Thomas N. Tallman

My darling son and friend—who tried to make others feel better even when he was so ill—who loved the sun and water and longed for the tropics—who had music as part of his being—and gave me the sun and song in my heart because he was my loved and loving son—who could make a plant flourish with his touch—but, like many blooms, has gone too soon

In loving remembrance,
Mark's Mom

LONNIE RICHARDS ═══════════════

I met Lonnie Richards in the unlikeliest of places to meet the love of your life. It was a late and loaded night at a small, dark bar in Silverlake. We cruised; we connected; we went home. It was like a lot of nights and yet immediately it was different.

It was afterwards, when I held him, that I first felt the glow. It was just a warm feeling, right in the center of my chest and then in the pit of my stomach. There was something there. This guy felt completely different.

As I came to know him, as we spent our days that became years together, the reasons became a lot clearer than they were that first mysterious, rather magical evening. Lonnie was a very bright man, to be sure; though he didn't wear his smarts on his sleeve, he had a degree in nuclear engineering from Texas A&M. He was an engineer for Exxon. He had strong, intelligent opinions and insights and was not afraid to share them.

But above all, he was perhaps the most innocent person I've ever known, and I think I felt instantly drawn to, and protective of, that quality. He could get angry, but he was really without malice. Decency was just basic with him . . .

I remember one time, shortly after we moved in together, a photo place called trying to sell him some portrait shots. He signed us up. When we wanted to be photographed together, the photographer asked, "What are you guys, brothers or something?" Without missing a beat, Lonnie just said, "No, we're gay, and we're lovers." Just like that, matter of fact.

He accepted himself utterly, and he accepted and loved me, just as I was. When he was diagnosed, he accepted that, too, and taught me how to live through it.

I miss him terribly and always will. I miss the dancing (he was a genuine cowboy, from Amarillo, Texas!), the talks, the wonderful trips together, the coming home every night to his words, his hugs, his understanding, his company.

But most of all, I miss that glow. From the first night, it never changed. I felt it when I held him all night, on the last night of his life.

Dave Johnson

We made this quilt all in one day, just the way Jeff liked to do things! He was so energetic and had such a positive attitude about everything. He took such good care of his body, it's hard to believe we lost him so quickly. There were so many more things to do, to experience; it was always too early for him to go home.

I miss Jeff. I knew him for enough years to have developed a very comfortable understanding; he was a permanent part of my life. I was looking forward to enjoying his friendship for many, many years.

Susan Sommerfeld

Like a white-winged dove,
He takes to the sky on his flight
Leaving behind
All his problems in the night.
Soaring to the tops
Of the clouds
Till Heaven Almighty he'll reach,
There he'll find happiness
In the Kingdom of Love,
And his problems will rest in peace.

My friend Kevin Murphy wrote those words several years ago. On December 13, 1990, at 33 years of age, Kevin leapt from his hospital window, ending his pain.

Kevin was a loving, gentle man who worked with handicapped people. He was a devoted father to his three children; he loved his family, his friends, and God.

Kevin possessed a beautiful singing voice and was a talented songwriter. He sang at my wedding just four years ago despite being ill. Kevin and I were "true friends" (his words) for 12 years. We confided in and comforted each other, and laughed and danced and worked together.

I miss you Kevin; you are forever in my heart.

Love to you, my buddy,
Lauri

May 13, 1991

MICHAEL APUZZO ════════════════════════

My brother Mike was born on July 20, 1959. It was on his tenth birthday that man first walked on the moon. That was a big day for Mickey, as we called him then; we were allowed to stay up that night and watch the first blurry black-and-white transmissions from the surface of the moon. We watched the planting of the American flag and the hitting of the first golf ball in outer space. Somehow the world seemed to be headed for great things, and Mickey's birthday was the mark of this bold new era. At night he and our mother would look at the stars through his telescope. He loved to look for Orion and the Big Dipper.

By July 20, 1979, his 20th birthday, we were calling him Mike. He was a student at Pratt Institute, one of the illustration department's rising stars. He was passionate about civil rights, gay rights and the poor children that lived in his neighborhood in Brooklyn. His paintings reflected the world as Mike saw it, depicting children holding knives or shooting drugs, along with more gentle works, a shyly smiling boy holding a basketball, a girl squeezing her dog.

By July 20, 1989, his 30th birthday, Mike was dead. He had graduated from Pratt, then gone to Hofstra Law School. In the law, he found a purposefulness in life that probably led to the happiness he seemed to exude during those years.

But who was Mike, really? He was a person without enemies, with more friends than anyone else I've ever known. He was the person that you called to help you paint your apartment, or feed your cats or make ten trays of lasagne for your sister's shower. He was there for everyone he loved, whenever they needed him. He could make a party out of one bottle of cheap wine and a bag of potato chips. He loved cartoons, he loved flowers, he loved Lucy and the *Honeymooners*.

He loved to do things, from exploring an old subway stop in Brooklyn to having his picture taken at Edgar Allan Poe's grave in Baltimore. He loved the theatre, and was a great organizer of events, from hot air ballooning to treasure hunts. He got locked in a New Orleans cemetery he was exploring during Mardi Gras. His secret ambition was to star in a Broadway musical.

When Mike first became ill, in November of 1987, he promised himself to fight to the bitter end. In June of 1988, he lost both sight and hearing in one week's time. He made a Helen Keller joke to his doctor.

For the last ten months of his life, though unable to see or hear, he came home and we spent our first summer together since college. He went to the beach, swam, made ice cream and tried to do the things that had always made summer special to him. As sick as he was, Mike was always fun to be around. He made us laugh and he made us cry . . .

I remember holding his hand moments before he died, and watching his fingers turn blue. And I knew then even though July 20, 1969 was in all the history books, July 20, 1959 was a much more important date.

Linda Apuzzo

EDDIE JAMES ANTHONY ═══════════

Eddie Anthony was a beautiful, lovely and lean black-haired man with big damp brown eyes and a wide handsome triangular nose like a munificent jack-o-lantern, well-lit from within. He died the day after Christmas '86, the tree blazing in front of him, at home with me. I continued to tear out the Sunday Times puzzle for many months after that although Eddie was no longer around to gnaw on his nails over that damn crossword. Although it's an over-roasted chestnut, it's true: I loved him more than life itself . . .

Eddie had several careers and was very concerned about the plight of the gay community for years before AIDS meant anything other than a chewy chocolatey diet candy supplement. When we met 12 years ago, he was a singer doing various gigs on cruise ships to Aruba and showcases at Upstairs at the Downstairs, Town Hall and Reno Sweeney's. He gave up his singing career, never looking back (as was his way), and founded two fundraising gay health organizations, the Robert Livingston Memorial Foundation and Gay Is Healthy, and produced several benefits at The Saint featuring Tina Turner and Grace Jones. (Three years ago we still had 500 t-shirts featuring the red, traffic-stopping logo "Gay Is Healthy" in our hall closet; don't think they were easy to unload in 1985!) . . .

One day six or eight years ago in some momentary fit of silly exuberance, I tossed a dime out the window. It hit the railing and fell onto the outside sill where it remained. I said to Eddie: "Don't touch that, it's our Love Dime." And that dime stayed out there, heads up, for years. Eddie's mother once tried to take it off the sill, it had gotten so discolored and dull. But Eddie told her, "Don't fool with that, it's our Love Dime." When he died and, against my better judgment, he was done up for a "viewing," the one thing I insisted on was that the funeral director place that Love Dime in Eddie's left hand . . . And that's just where it went. I know Eddie would have liked that.

Kerry Kammer

Jerry "Bud" Mullen, Jr.

Jerry was born in Long Beach, California (1959), and moved to Sweet Home, Oregon (1971), where he graduated from high school (1977).

Jerry started working in grocery stores at age 15. He moved to Las Vegas, Nevada (1980), and was employed with Lucky Markets until he became ill (1987).

Jerry's first love was his family, and his main interest was stock car racing. At age 17, he had his own race car, #29, and raced the 1976 season in Lebanon, Oregon, winning Rookie Driver of the Year.

When Jerry was just a child, he and his sister would sing songs at bedtime. The Johnny Appleseed song was his favorite. They sang it together some hours before his passing.

He also loved flowers, music, and his cat "Macho." All the things he loved most are included on his quilt panel, which was made by his family.

Jerry had many friends and was always willing to help anyone, in any way he could. He was a good person, a kind and loving son and brother. We were always very proud of him and we will always love and miss him. He made our little family complete.

Mom and Dad,
sister Candace,
brother Monte

This panel was made for Chad Andrew Henry, who was, and always shall be, my dearest friend. It was made by myself and by his much-loved sister, Claudia Davis. The quilt speaks to the importance of friendship and love in Chad's life and to the comfort, peace, and assurance he found in his faith as a Christian.

He was 26-and-a-half and one day old when he died in Sacramento, California, on April 26, 1991. He died surrounded by family and dear friends, and he was sent out from this world knowing that he was much loved. He will *never* be forgotten. The brilliant light of his life shall always illuminate that place in our hearts that is his to live in forever.

*Ray Freer and
Claudia Davis*

13 months and 8 days as recorded in Earth time, you were with us. But you will live in our memories forever. You were not born, nor did you pass, in vain.

The lives that you touched are all better for having known you. The incredible strength from one so small, who endured physical pain beyond the ability to scream, is bravery and courage we can only guess at. Your eyes always told the story. You could not speak, but your message was, and is still being heard. We will be your voice.

On this day, when your square takes its place with the rest who have passed with you, on the great Quilt, it is a tribute to you, my darling Tati Angel. You were, and still are, our very special gift. You taught us well. Although we are separated from you in the present moment, we are always one in spirit.

Till we meet again, your family:

Mom, Dad, Carolee Vogel, Bruce, your sisters, Marisa and Arianna, your brothers, Junior and Jeremy

April 27, 1990

I made this quilt piece for C.J. The quilt does not bear his name because his family does not want anyone to know their son died of AIDS.

I met C.J. a month before he died. I visited him every day until he died. He struggled a great deal and knew of his family's struggle to accept him and the fact that he had AIDS. The saying on the quilt piece, "I Love You a Skyful" is one his mother chose when I told her I wanted to do a piece for the Quilt. It is what she used to say to him from the time he was a little boy.

It was my hope that seeing this as part of the NAMES Quilt she would be able to grieve openly with others who have had loved ones [who have] died of AIDS.

That has not happened yet. I have hope it will. Until then, I celebrate the life of this wonderful gay man with this panel sewn in love.

Kay

WALT A. ═══════════════════════════

Our relationship with Walt was pretty simple. Walt was the official scorekeeper of our gay softball team, The Brass Rail Rebels of Minneapolis, Minnesota . . .

A few stories: Walt was the official scorer and he was tough. You really had to earn your base hits. On several occasions team members would be batting for the batting title and Walt would be stingy and call possible base hits errors. Hence the question "That was a hit, wasn't it, Walt?"

The question would always lead to a wonderful response. Either a nod or a shake of the head, possibly a slight smile, and then a swig of mineral water . . .

Walt kept his life to himself. We didn't know a lot about his life away from softball, but it really didn't matter. He was always there for us. Whether we were playing in Minneapolis, Milwaukee, or Kansas City, Walt was there. Don't sit on the end of the bench because that's Walt's spot.

The last time I was with Walt was in San Francisco at the gay softball World Series of 1987. We stood together cheering on our archrival Twin Cities team, the Cloud Nine Americans, to the championship.

I know Walt was happy to see them win even though we both knew they could never possess the true love and dedication for each other that our team has.

Walt left us quickly. I was out of town in January 1988 when Walt died. I missed the memorial service and that has left an empty feeling in me. Making this panel has filled that empty space. The background is our team's original "Brass Rail" banner. Since we knew it would never be the same again without Walt we decided to give our team banner to him in the form of a panel for the Quilt.

Walt is in the action picture in his usual spot on the bench keeping score. In the team picture he is in the last row, right side. Many of his softball friends signed the left side of the panel. He didn't play the game but he was just as important to the team as any double-play or home run. Our lives will never be the same.

Walt—we love you, we miss you. Our dear friend, we will never forget.

That was a hit, wasn't it, Walt?

Greg Boorsma

Mark was 41 when he died September 3, 1986. He was 29 when we met—we had 12 years of growing and playing together—we attempted to storm adulthood together—sometimes, I wish we were kids again! . . .

Mark was raised by fundamentalist Christian ministers for parents and he spent his life dealing with their disapproval of his life. Before he died—a couple of years before—he realized that they wouldn't change—that *he* had to—and he did. He was beginning to see how much he was loved . . . his friends were for life!

I wanted a show piece, a piece that would stand against all the anger and denial of his person—his spirit—his sexuality—his dying that his parents bombarded him with—I wanted a thing of beauty to shine for my friend with the talent that I have—my art and my heart—I wanted a final testimonial that Mark was loved . . .

And I wanted to say goodbye.

Patrick Shapard

I made this panel for a friend and my buddy. Mark was matched with me through the buddy system. We were together for four months before he died. Mark was a person who enjoyed the finer things in life: clothes, food and above all, chocolate.

He developed toxoplasmosis rapidly and lost the intelligence that he was very proud of. His love of chocolate was not lost. Many of his days in the hospital were spent eating chocolate.

About a week after the Quilt had been displayed in Oklahoma City, he developed N.P. They said that Mark would only have a few days to live. On one of those days I went to relieve his mom for awhile. Mark was sitting up in bed eating chocolate. He had chocolate from ear to ear. Mark motioned for me to come over to his hospital bed. Barely able to speak, he said, "Thank you, Rod," and then pulled me down closer and gave me a kiss on the cheek, then said "I love you!"

As I rose up from his bed, he started laughing at the chocolate on my face. A week later Mark died. I miss him.

Rod Limke

AL J.

Our son Al was the oldest of our three children. I could sit down and write him up to be a "saint," but he was not. I will say he was a very loving and caring person who touched the lives of all who came in touch with him. He had a very dry sense of humor, but you always knew where you stood with him.

Al had been on his own since about his 18th birthday, college, the Navy and then on to California to "find himself." Coming from a small community, the mere mention of being gay was taboo, and he felt he did not want to hurt his loved ones with his way of life.

His brother Mike and he as youngsters did not get along very well, but as young men and becoming more mature their love for each other grew like no other love could for two brothers. Mike now is bitter over the fact that he no longer has his brother to share his life and his experiences . . .

Al's sister Maria never got to know him too well, as there was 11 years' difference, but the last two years of Al's life, she was starting to get to know him.

Al was so looking forward to Maria's wedding, but his life ended almost three months before the wedding. We, his parents, how can we describe the loss we feel, knowing we'll never hear his voice, sharing holidays or just a visit to spend some time together. Our grateful feeling is knowing he knew we loved him and always supported him in his life, and will always have him in our hearts in our lifetime.

Now we speak of Al's lover, "Shermsie," as he called him. A delight to know, and we felt a close bond from the very moment we met him. Al felt his life was finally complete. The love and care "Sherms" gave Al during his most trying moments of his life is something one just cannot imagine. I wonder if I, his mother, could have handled it as well. I really think not. "Sherms" kept us informed constantly, and we are all grateful for him and feel we now have another son, whose love we'll always hold dear.

Al, we love and miss you.

Mom, Dad, Mike, Maria,
Becky and Shermsie

CURTIS A. MCMILLAN

We were given the opportunity to meet—and come to know and love Curtis and his family—through the pediatric program of GMHC. We met the McMillans in February 1986, shortly after Curtis' diagnosis of AIDS.

In addition to having AIDS, Curtis was also mentally retarded and suffered from cerebral palsy. Although he was nearly six years old when we met him, he was no bigger than a two-year-old and had none of the skills of a typical six-year-old. His communications skills were rudimentary at the best of times, and he was only able to walk, when he was strong, with the use of a walker. He required diapers and often needed help feeding himself.

Yet, despite his many handicaps, Curtis was a friendly, inquisitive boy with a brilliant smile. He enjoyed his toys, going for rides in his wheelchair around the neighborhood and the attention of his family and friends. His favorite toy was an old wig of his mother's which he would play with for hours.

Curtis was fortunate that he was surrounded by his loving adoptive mother and his caring brother and sisters, as well as many friends.

We feel very lucky having known this very special little boy and his family. Though it is perhaps lacking in creative genius, the panel we created in memory of Curtis does show how much we loved this most special person—and how much we miss him.

*Alan Levine and
Julie Ritzer Russ*

. . . I cried when I heard Billy was diagnosed, and Dallas promised to give me Billy's address so I could write to him.

Two weeks later when I asked Dallas for the address, he started to cry, and I knew that a letter was too late. We clung to each other and cried—more than we had ever laughed.

Billy was my first friend to die of AIDS. Dallas is sick now and I don't know how many more panels I will have to make . . .

Nancy Blanford

To ALL THE CHILDREN WHO HAVE AIDS,
TO ALL THE CHILDREN WHO HAVE DIED OF
AIDS

We are the Camp Fire Boys and Girls in the 4th grade. We made this quilt for you because we want you to know that we care.

Our hand prints symbolize that we are reaching out to help and love you. We hope that this quilt will remind all the adults that we, the children, are the future of tomorrow. We should not be forgotten or ignored because we are smaller than you.

We hope when this quilt travels across the country, all the love we put into making it will spread the message of hope and peace to everyone that touches it!

Love always,

Santa Clara/Santa Cruz Counties
Council of Camp Fire Boys and Girls

May 19, 1989

Although I had known Tim for five years, I did not realize how well I knew him until after he had died. Tim and I met in a very unique way when I was 15 years old. After seeing "Cats," I decided that I wanted to meet the man who performed the role of Mr. Mistoffeles. My friend and I discussed the ways we might meet Tim. Originally, we contacted the press representatives for the show and requested an interview . . . We said we were writing an article for our high school newspaper. While they agreed to grant us the interview, they never followed through with any of their promises to arrange it. Taking the initiative, I figured it would not hurt to try calling Tim at home.

We discovered that Tim's phone number was listed in the phone book and called him. I was so nervous. When he answered, I told him who I was and explained that I wanted to do an interview with him. Tim agreed and suggested that we meet at the theater. I was overwhelmed. We wrote questions (most of which were foolish, looking back on them now) and went to the interview. No matter how silly the question, Tim answered and explained to us. I learned so much about theater by just talking to him and asking questions. He was so helpful and patient.

That interview was the beginning of a special relationship I had with Tim. Through phone calls, mini-interviews for some real research papers I did in school, and lunches, I came to know Tim and was

continued

introduced to his positive philosophy of life. . . . Now
. . . his death.

On January 5, 1985, Tim and I had lunch. That
was the last time I ever saw him. He toured with Chita
Rivera and moved to Los Angeles. When I entered
college, I lost touch with him. I always knew, in the
back of my mind, that we would meet up again.
During our lunch, Tim and I had discussed my plans
for the future. He encouraged me to become a talent
agent . . . He continued by saying that he would want
me to be his agent, when I finally made it. Boy, was
that a boost of confidence! . . . Since then, I've been
doing everything I can to be the kind of agent Tim
thought I could be . . . I may be a peon now, but
eventually things have to get better . . . Then I'll be an
agent!

Last September, I spoke with a friend of mine
who recently became a dresser for "Cats" . . . She
mentioned to me that people in the cast were upset
because they had heard that the original Mistoffeles
had AIDS. I asked her the name of the performer,
praying that it wasn't Tim, even though I had known

that Tim was the original Mistoffeles. She said his name was Scott something. "Timothy Scott," I asked. She said yes. My heart sunk . . . A week later I called him on his 32nd birthday. He was happy to hear from me, but he sounded so weak . . .

Because I did not see Tim suffer with AIDS, I really do not have any concept of the pain that he went through. The media has given me an idea of what happens to a person who has AIDS. I cannot imagine Tim having to suffer like that . . . No one should have to suffer with AIDS.

I'm sure that everyone who has made panels for members of their families and/or friends, feels as strongly as I do. The love and time put into each stitch is just a small indication of what these loved ones mean to us . . . Tim, you're in a better place now . . . I just miss you so much. Enjoy your next Jellicle life and stay as special as you are. I hope we meet again.

I love you!

Wendy K. Wetstein

August 4, 1988

Dear Friends,

Herewith I send you my personal panel for the Quilt project. It contains the names of the 39 people with AIDS who asked me to walk with them in their last days.

I am a Franciscan priest and co-founder of Project Lazarus, Louisiana's only residence for people with AIDS . . . Doing this work and living in the French Quarter, I was made aware of the illness about five years ago, but at that time it was very hush-hush—"Oh, he died of pneumonia . . ." I began to realize that more and more people were getting sick and in deeper need. Finally a friend told me of a guy at Charity Hospital with AIDS due to be released and homeless, and "Could I help?" . . .

After four years of intense involvement in the AIDS crisis in various roles, I decided to step aside for a year and a half and take a sabbatical. I am afraid that we are in this for a long haul—I do not want to be burned out. While in Chicago on sabbatical, the Quilt came to town—I volunteered to work on the Quilt as a grief counsellor. My work on the Quilt helped me get in touch with my own grief. I needed to express publicly my love and grief for the men and women I have walked with, wept with and loved who have died—and who are dying . . .

Thank you for offering this opportunity to me for making memory of these men and women who have so blessed my life—knowing them and receiving their love has changed me radically. For a long time, I hestitated in making a panel. After all, I thought, I was not their next of kin, blood brother or lover. I felt that I had to bear my tears alone for these who I have loved and who have loved me.

After viewing the Quilt, I have realized that in every fact I was and am: THEIR NEXT OF KIN, THEIR BROTHER AND LOVER and that this panel belongs with all those other panels in the Quilt.

Thank you,

Rev. Bob Pawell, O.F.M.

September 2, 1991

This letter was written by Brent Nicholson Earle, who ran across the United States to raise money for AIDS research, in memory of his friends Court Miller, Jim Johnson, David Summers, Jimmy Roddy, Bill McTarnahan, Paul Popham, Frank DiGennaro, Fritz Holt, Dr. Tom Waddell, Ignacio Zuazo, David Lee and Ken Gelow.

I think that writing these memorials is one of the hardest things I've ever had to do, harder even than all of the miles I ran around America. I believe that one of the reasons I've had such a difficult time is that, although these memorials will become part of public record, I need to say what these people meant to me personally.

Hearing some of the memorials read aloud at the Kennedy Center during the Quilt's return to Washington has helped to give me courage to follow the path of my heart. Yet still I've had to deal with a lot of resistance within myself to finishing them. Perhaps I feel that once I've sent them off, I will have finally let go. And part of me desperately wants to hold on . . .

Sadly, our loss is much greater than just these 14 friends. So many other dear friends lie in honor within the Quilt, and many more have yet to be remembered there. Having recently received the confirmation of my own HIV positivity, I can't help but wonder if I, too, will one day find a place of rest there among my comrades . . .

With gratitude and love,

Brent Nicholson Earle
for the American Run
for the End of AIDS

July 30, 1989

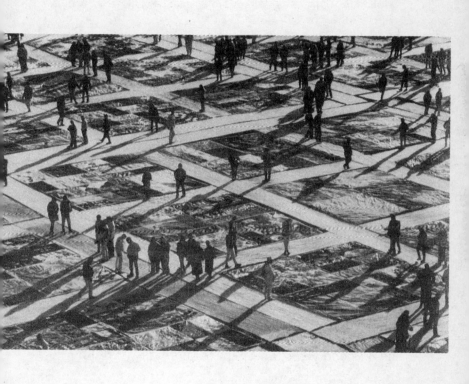

Bruce wanted to leave us quietly today, but I could not let him go without telling the world how much I loved him. He was my brother, my childhood playmate, and, most important, my best friend.

Bruce walked through life giving of himself to others. He was always there with a kind word and a helping hand. He was a man of love.

Through his illness, I think Bruce brought out the best in us. Now it was our turn to do for him, and we were all able to care for him with the same loyalty and love that he gave to us.

Bruce was able to accept his illness with courage. In the beginning, he seemed to sense that we needed the comforting. When I cried because the thought of losing him seemed unbearable, he put his arms around me and hugged me and said, "It's okay to cry, Karlen." When a friend questioned the fact that he would be taken from us so soon, he reminded us that none of us were promised anything. He said, "I have had 42 good years, and I am ready to die." I think it was his gentle way of telling each of us to take a good look at our own lives to make sure that we are getting the most out of each and every day, so that when our time comes to die, we, too, can say, "I have had so many good years."

I try not to look on today as a day of sadness, because I truly believe Bruce is singing with the angels and sitting at the right hand of God. I ask each of you not to wish him back: Be happy for him, carry him forever in your hearts, and be grateful that he touched our lives.

Bruce and I have traveled full circle together, from his birth to his death, and it was an experience in life that I shall never have again, so I consider it to have been a very special gift. Bruce has been such a part of my life that he will never be gone from me. He was a giver, and when he was very sick, he made a very special promise to me. So Bruce, wherever you are, watch over me and continue to love me.

Karlen Pitzka-Urban

JANICE BERMAN

Janice Berman was our mother and our best friend. Her capacity for love and giving was infinite; her intellect, superior. She was a quiet non-conformist who set her own standards. She could always make us laugh.

Sometimes we laughed for joy, and sometimes to keep from crying. She once said she laughed her way from hospital room to hospital room. And it was true. There were too many hospital rooms and too much hardship in our mom's life—particularly in the last few years, when both she and our dad suffered from a series of illnesses. But she never complained. She made the best of what life gave her.

Janice grew up in Brooklyn, the youngest of six daughters, raised by a widowed mother. As a young woman, she developed her lifelong interest in politics and social justice. We can remember her telling how she worked on the unsuccessful campaign to save Julius and Ethel Rosenberg from the electric chair. And many years and many unpopular causes later, we remember how, on the night George McGovern lost, she comforted us, especially her eldest child, an idealistic 17-year-old, by singing "Our Day Will Come" . . .

She was the kind of mother who would share with a three-year-old the pictures in a book of Rembrandts; the kind of mother who would stay up late typing a term paper for a procrastinating teenager; the kind of mother, wife and adventurous spirit who would set off for a cross-country trip in a camper—with an eight-year-old, a four-year-old, and a two-year-old (on later trips we would add a cat) . . .

Our mother Janice Berman was infected with the AIDS virus through blood transfusions she received during hip replacement surgery. She was diagnosed with pneumocystis pneumonia in March 1987. Four months later, our father died after suffering a second stroke. Our mom lived only six months after dad's death. She died January 12, 1988 –at the age of 56.

The last years of our mother's life were full of painful events—events that still dominate our memories. But we try to remember—she lived a life full of love, love both given and received. We had good times together, and she taught us how to make the bad times as good as they could be . . .

We miss her every day.

Karen, Robert and
Ellen Berman

In April of 1990, our congregation held a weekend-long symposia on AIDS in the Jewish community. During that time we hosted a section of the Quilt at our synagogue. The impact of the Quilt was so great that members of our congregation created these panels for their loved ones who died from this disease.

The three individuals for whom the panels are dedicated are named on the cloth. Their backgrounds remain a mystery other than that which is depicted on the panels.

All these people were Jewish and are related to members of our congregation. Our hope is that you will add these panels to an existing section and that one day we may bring this panel back to Milwaukee.

Thank you for your help when it was needed and now as well . . .

Rabbi David A. Lipper and Congregation Emanu-El B'ne Jeshurun

This panel is for David Michael Rolland. He was my son and my best friend.

David was only 23 when he was diagnosed; he was really just coming into his life. He moved to Berkeley, California, to live with me when he became unable to work in 1986. For two and one half years, we lived as though on our own planet, trying to have as much as possible, trying to ride the waves of this merciless disease. We had a lot of help along the way from loving friends. Many came into our lives when the struggle was the most desperate and we were the most battered by the storm. Three of these friends helped me to design and make this panel.

David was a New Yorker . . . he thought California was part of the Ice Age. He never would have moved here by choice. We are very glad he did. We loved him, hurt with him, hoped and cried with him. We were awed by his diversity, inspired by the depth of his honor and dignity and amused and enlightened as well. A light has gone out in our lives and an ache has replaced it that cannot be pacified.

The panel speaks best for what David was . . . having it become part of the larger Quilt is in a way another loss, but we want to bear witness.

It is my hope that every panel becomes a person to every person who still believes AIDS is not their concern.

Thank you all for bearing witness.
Susan M. Black

This panel I am submitting to you is for a young man that I came to know for only 38 days. His name was Byron and we did not meet as most friends do. I call it an "arranged" friendship. We were matched up as buddies in Project Ahead (Long Beach Area) Buddy Program.

When I met Byron, I was not sure what to expect. I was told that he was very thin, so I prepared myself. Well, I arrived at the board and care home where he was staying at our prearranged time and found him asleep . . . I wasn't aware of the fact that he was on medication and the effects it had on him . . . I did not realize how much the drug took out of him and how weak he would become.

Byron was very strong-willed and wanted his environment a certain way. I guess he felt that was one thing he could control—his surroundings. I would often put up pictures he had cut out of *National Geographics* on his walls but most of our time was spent silently.

I did most of the talking. I used to get angry because I was the one talking all the time, telling him about my day, my family and whatever I could come up with. I'd ask him about his day . . . but his responses seemed very brief. I realize now that for whatever reason, he couldn't talk to me. I don't know if he didn't trust me. But I learned to respect his privacy. I wish, though, that he would have told me his favorite color.

Byron died on June 4, 1989. That also happens to

be my father's birthday. I thought about people being born and dying every day. I did not find out until the 6th of June when I called to see how he was doing. We'd sometimes go a few days without seeing each other, and although I knew his condition had worsened, I did not know how far along he was. No one had bothered to call me. I wish I could have been there with him but I was also told that he died peacefully in his sleep.

There was no memorial service for Byron. His family chose not to have one. On June 15, 1989, I had a ceremony for Byron by myself . . . I bought three helium-filled balloons (to represent him, me, and our friendship), went to a park in Long Beach that overlooked the ocean and wrote him a letter. In that letter I wrote my feelings about this relationship that we had in the previous five and a half weeks. I wrote of my anger and frustration, and of my growing and coming to a place of peace. I wrote of those things I wished he had shared with me and of how much I felt we had communicated through the silence. And I wrote how much of an impact he had on my life in that short period and wondered if there was snow where he was. He had never been to the snow.

After I finished the letter, I tied it to the balloons and let it go. I thought "Maybe he'll be able to read it." Kind of corny, I guess. It's funny but I was hoping that it would fly out over the ocean but the wind took it back over into the city. I guess that was more appropriate. He was a city kid.

Daniel Calma

Harry W. Adams, Jr.

What a heartbreaking day it was when our only brother, who we loved dearly, died from AIDS! Harry was a warm, loving, gifted, generous man and we and his many, many friends whose lives he touched will always miss him sorely.

All of us girls eventually left home to get married but he stayed with Mom and Dad, and when they were old he saw to it that they had the best of everything and wanted for nothing. They never knew the agony of being alone and afraid of their future . . .

How much we wish that he had come back to St. Louis where we could have cared for him in his last days. Harry never told us he was gay but we knew it from his lifestyle. We should have been able to talk about it—it would have helped all of us. We didn't know he had AIDS until about 18 months before he died . . .

We have made his panel for the Quilt with a Christmas theme. Everyone who knew Harry knew what Christmas meant to him. Harry was constantly buying tree ornaments all year long. He had trains set on a platform on which stood the tree and a tiny village. He even bought a beautiful imported nativity set which we cherish.

This is our memorial to our brother Harry from his sisters, brothers-in-law, nephews, nieces and friends . . .

Harry, we love you. Save a place for us and one day we will all be together again.

Catherine (Mickey) Phillips

What can I say . . . He died in late summer of '84. He was living in L.A. at the time, me in S.F.

Martin (though my nickname for him was Juji, coined from the Jujifruit candies) was mostly Jewish, and guilt kept us together as best buddies. In fact, Martin used to say "There's not enough guilt in the world."

He was sarcastic, wild, loved the gym, leather and wanted to be successful someday in his writings. Somewhere in L.A. is a novel, half-finished. I read each page as it came from the typewriter.

Near the end . . . we had a horrible fight. Actually, he did. I just listened.

Though I never got to say goodbye, I'll never forget my last words to him: "I'm sorry you feel this way, but I love you."

Gary D'Alois

I never knew Susan Roggio.

When I lead AIDS prevention discussions for teens, I show a videotape that features three PWAs talking about their lives, their illness, and their wishes for a legacy of AIDS prevention among youth. Susan Roggio is one of them.

She is beautiful and bold and brave, and she breaks my heart.

This woman beat drug addiction and rebuilt her life. Every time I see the tape, I feel cheated not to have known her. I feel cheated that the world never got to know her children.

When the NAMES Project came to town, I called Bill B., the AIDS volunteer coordinator where I worked, to see if she had been remembered with a panel. He called me back at 5:10 p.m. this Thursday evening. We talked about what a lovely woman she seemed to be, and what kind of panel might suit her.

It was the last I ever spoke with him. Bill went

home and died that same evening, due to complications of AIDS.

Susan's panel became a group project. My friend, Gail Hedberg, did much of the sewing. Another friend, Alisa Shapiro, assisted with the design and enlisted the help of a colleague to design the lettering. (When he gave her the completed stencils, she said, "Thanks, I owe you one." He replied: "Thank *you*. My brother just died of AIDS.")

As you can see, there are a lot of emotions tied up with this panel, and several others besides Susan whom it indirectly honors.

We chose the color combination of black and white for its beauty and its stark representation of life and death. We felt the vibrant, free-form flowers suited Susan's personality. We hope, wherever she is now, that she is just as free. We pray for a cure.

Sincerely,

Linda Haase

Steven Bailey fell ill to AIDS very early (1983–84) when AIDS was not fully understood and when treatment and doctors were not . . . well informed. Consequently, he suffered an awful lot and when he was hospitalized, prejudice was very prevalent.

But Steve was a very brave and courageous young man.

Far too many friends and relatives were hesitant to visit him and it broke our hearts. He chose to die in his home with nurses around the clock to avoid the prejudices he received in the hospital.

Steve was a very handsome dapper man who always dressed very well. His ties on the quilt depict his good taste in his appearance. He loved Cadillacs and had five in his happy life, therefore the Cad panel on the quilt . . . also he had a miniature schnauzer, Zeta, who was his pride and joy and laid by his side and on his bed during his long illness. He enjoyed her so much and therefore the dog panel on the quilt depicts his love for his dog.

The quilt shows just a small part of his happy, generous love of live. He left a loving and understanding Mom and Dad and many good friends.

Your loving parents,
Charles and Dorothy Bailey

I met Brian while he was a patient in the hospital. I am an R.N.

Brian was a very private person and the reason we got to be friends was he had basically shut out the world and we started talking. He felt he could talk to me because I already knew his diagnosis. His brothers and mother had been told he was HIV positive just the Christmas before. As far as I know his friends and other family members never knew he was sick . . .

His family doesn't know that I'm doing this. It was something I wanted to do for him . . .

Brian came from Coon Valley, Wisconsin, and he loved Davy Crockett. His Davy Crockett cap was one of his prized possessions; so I have included a raccoon in the quilt square. Brian was an attorney for the government—Wild Life Division. Toward the end he played a song "In The Garden" over and over again, so the garden is a special part of his quilt . . .

I have taken care of a lot of HIV+ and AIDS patients. Brian was the first one that I became very close to as he reminded me a lot of my late husband. My family had to keep reminding me that I was already widowed and was not going to be widowed again when Brian died. It was a hard time for all of us.

It was interesting—Brian's father had died about five years ago and his mother had taken care of him at home also—I asked her once if it was harder to lose a husband or a son and she told me it was harder to lose a son.

D. M.

This quilt bearing 30 names is in memory of the staff and members of "The Saint."

This disco, which opened its doors in September 1980, was the most expensive wholly gay enterprise in the U.S. and cost in excess of 4.5 million dollars. It originally operated as a gay membership disco, open only Saturday and Sunday nights and legally held 3,224 in its 40,000 square feet on three levels. Opening year, it boasted four female members and 3,220 men . . . members hailed from all 50 states and more than 20 countries. In all, prior to closing on May 2, 1988 with a 56-hour non-stop party, it saw over 174 million men pass through its glass and bronze doors on Saturdays and Sundays.

To explain the quilt is simple: the silver bar at the bottom reading "Hold On To My Love" was the last song played at the club's closing, prior to the two-hour classical music requiem mass. The red section represents the "dome" or heart of the club. The dance space was circular with four entry portals and with banquettes. The "tree" in the center of the dance floor held over 500 lights plus the machine which produced this effect plus various special effects. The entire tree was on hydraulics so that direction and intensity could be instantaneously changed. The star machine was the single most expensive piece of equipment in the club. The mirrored ball entered and left the dome via a trap door in the dome . . .

The black area is the unknown: The silver shafts of energy many claim to have seen, others felt generated in the club. Each shaft bears (or unfortunately will have) the name of a member who has gone over to dance under an eternal dome, since like the Saint, they no longer exist except in our memories.

The Saint was a place to go, meet friends, party

and make new friends; but it was more—it was an expanded family. It was a place, once experienced, one will not forget. Likewise, the experience of having had some of these people as friends and lovers will remain with us as long as we have life.

Tony played the lights to the crowd, seeming to know where all heads were simultaneously at, while Shaun geared the music to each person's head and yet all heads. Michael worked his fans, sometimes as many as six at once on the stage, banquettes or just as frequently on the mezzanine.

Kanghi saw that everyone had their supplies, so as to design their inner selves and heads. Magioncalda kept his shorts, even in winter, drying on the locker room radiator. Meanwhile, Noseworthy saw to it that all guests were admitted as per a member's request and that our locker room's security was never breached. Mario labored in his studio to create fantastic visual effects such as E.T.'s finger coming up to touch the ball, which then began to glow. To silhouette hundreds of hot, naked men dancing for a black party, or every pill, capsule, powder and designer drug known to be projected on the dome to the strains of "White Rabbit" for a white party. Tommy inspired his lover to create what many professional publications consider the best-designed and executed dance club, bar none. From bathrooms with angled mirrors to a 1,500 lb. slab of poured concrete to stabilize the turntables, he left nothing to chance.

Such were the members and staff of the Saint, to which many owe thanks, and all who went have "Memories"—a song Betty Buckley once sang upon the stage, costume and all . . .

Mary E. Nesnick, member

This panel is for a man called Steven Fields. I pray I'll never have to do another one . . .

Who is Steve Fields? That's a hard question. Steven only came into my life three years ago. He was a friend of my lover at the time. He was a bartender with a heart of gold, though by no means was he a saint.

My friendship with Steven grew when we had a common interest: country dancing. He was good. Damn good. It was a pleasure to waltz with him. He later took that love of country further and bought himself a horse, Maria. He even went as far as to enter the Los Angeles Gay Rodeo. We were all so proud.

Steve had a teddy bear quality about him. He loved to hug and be hugged. It was easy to like him.

Steve kept it quiet about having AIDS down to his last week in the hospital. Most of his friends were not even told he was there until a week before he died. His death was quick and, I pray, painless.

He made a point of hanging around to say goodbye to everyone. At his funeral, his family ignored the fact that he died of AIDS and ignored his gay friends. Most of us were very angry because we never got a chance to say goodbye. The service was solemn and depressing. Steve was a party animal. He never thought of tomorrow or the consequences.

So, after the service, I suggested making the panel.

Little did I know of all the work involved. After talking to you guys at the NAMES Project, I felt better and thought I could pull it off. It took over two months of planning but it finally happened. There were a lot of tears but also a lot of laughing. Everyone sewed on the panel whether they knew how or not.

I even spilled some of my blood on there when I pricked my finger. I was never cut out to be Donna Reed.

I was a friend to Steve Fields. We only saw each other every couple of months, but there was always love . . .

With much love,
Michael Witt

I met a man in a bar several months ago who had lost several friends two years ago and has been running ever since looking for a place where no one is dying of AIDS—he hadn't started to grieve—he had run out of places to run—he was and is in pain.

Because of that chance meeting (is anything by chance?) I chose to organize a healing space and make this panel.

I designed it based on the first verse of the 137th Psalm:

"By the waters of Babylon we sat down and wept, when we remembered you, O Zion."

Carolyn and I cut it out on her living room floor one night and Brother Andrew stitched it together. The names were added at the healing space and placed under the "waters of Babylon" are other remembrances.

We remember,

Br. Karl Welsher, LBC-F

Melvin Leigh "Jerry" Herbel

Jerry was born January 1, 1955, in Scotts Bluff, Nebraska. He lived briefly in Tennessee and other places before moving to Phoenix in November 1976, when he became my roommate and best friend. He stood about 5'8" tall, had brown hair and eyes, a beautiful smile, and a kind, loving personality. He also had a striking, muscular body and a finely honed, offbeat sense of humor. Jerry loved to salvage neon tubes from old signs and light them up in the garage at night. He loved working in the garden, and was especially fascinated by desert plants. Many times he would sit up late at night to watch the slow-motion opening of a night-blooming cactus and to smell its overpowering, if brief, perfume.

In constructing Jerry's NAMES Quilt, his lover, David Zeigler, and I chose to depict the Arizona desert at night, with authentic embroidered reproductions of native plants in full bloom. The landscape features silhouettes of Pinnacle Peak, the Mogollon Rim, Squaw Peak, Camelback Mountain, Weaver's Needle, and the Superstitions, as well as the states of Arizona and Nebraska. The stars in the sky depict actual constellations, which correctly locate a star named after Jerry, one year after his death from a systemic infection, resulting from AIDS, on August 10, 1985.

With the help of our friend Calvin Fjelstul, David and I constructed this Quilt in 1987. I took it to the March on Washington and carried it in the parade past the national Quilt, but chose not to donate it at that time. Now, in September of 1991, David and I have at last agreed to "let it go," so that others may enjoy it and learn a little about our wonderful friend Jerry.

Robert W. Severance

Shortly after Robb was ordained, he came to talk to me about difficulties he was having with being gay. He had been given my name by someone. For many of his years as a priest, Robb had a hard time, having been assigned to live with difficult people who did not understand or appreciate him. Fortunately, in his last couple years, . . . he was sent to a parish where he was loved and appreciated by his pastor and others.

In the last conversation that I had with Robb, a phone conversation a few weeks before he died, he told me of difficulties he was having with AIDS and with bad reactions he was having to the medications he was on.

Robb in a sense took over my place at the counseling agency. I was the priest on the staff. He became a counselor there shortly after I left the agency and the priesthood.

Robb's panel was made by Bernie Scholemer, his pastor; Pat Wibbenmeyer, his boss; Jardi Schmalz, a co-worker; Marion Hebrank, a worker at Most Precious Blood Parish; a priest friend; and myself. His name is spelled out with a stole used at his first Mass. The runner on the R is from a marathon race T-shirt given him by a friend. The heart stands for his compassion as a counselor. The white rose is a flower he loved. Pink was one of his favorite colors. The stole separating his name from his dates was one of his. The first date, made out of a tennis shoelace, is his birth year. A note comes next, because he loved music. The second date is the year of his ordination. The pink triangle between the second and third date is a tribute to his gayness. The final date is the year of his death.

John P. Hilgeman

The quilt enclosed was made in memory of James Nathan Scott, Jimmy to those of us who knew and loved him. He was my lover, confidant and friend.

When Jimmy and I first heard that he was HIV-positive, we were like so many gay couples in that we took our love and relationship very much for granted. Through our living with AIDS together and our fight for a normal life together, our love grew and matured. I have never felt such love from another person. I feel that even though Jimmy and I have been separated by death that I have been truly blessed. To be loved in such a way and to be able to give love with such happiness and devotion is the greatest gift I have ever received. My time left on Earth may not be long but I have never felt more prepared to live than I am now. It is for this that AIDS, in contrast to its victims, has provided me a life anew.

I will always miss Jimmy, but if ever death is swallowed up in victory, then his truly was . . .

Tom Barrett

July 31, 1991

Paul was new to Portland when we met in November 1987, but he was not new to AIDS. A full five years earlier, he discovered he was seropositive when he was diagnosed with PCP. Paul had signed up for a support group for diagnosed men that I was co-facilitating under the auspices of the Cascade AIDS Project (CAP). He and I developed a telephone relationship because he was a chronic non-attender and he was on my list for outreach. Later we joked about why he ever signed up for a group because he was definitely not a "group person." We decided it was obviously the vehicle that was meant to bring us together.

Paul lived alone when we first met and soon I was doing his laundry and grocery shopping because he was no longer able to do those tasks for himself. We were also spending many hours drinking coffee in his kitchen, realizing how much we had in common. Paul had a wonderful, loving relationship with his Aunt Jeanne, who called him from New York almost every day. On one infamous day, Paul said, "I was talking to Aunt Jeanne today, and I told her that if I wasn't gay and I didn't have AIDS, I'd want to marry you and live with you forever." It was one of those rare moments that becomes flash-frozen in time. I remember looking at him and saying, "Is that a problem for you?"

A week later he moved in with me and proposed. We postponed the official marriage because he was afraid he might lose his benefits and he was concerned about leaving me with debts, but from that point on we were in a committed relationship.

About a month before he died, he began talking about wanting to be married in a religious ceremony. He shared that idea with Fr. Gary McGinnis, his wonderful, loving spiritual advisor. Fr. Gary stood by "on call" waiting until Paul had a good day. He rushed over on the morning of August 9, 1990, and performed a short, but moving ceremony that meant a great deal to both of us.

We always hoped that a cure would be found and that we would be able to grow old together. Paul once said that if we could just have three years together he would be a happy man. We were just three months short of that goal . . . When he realized death was inevitable, Paul wanted to meet it on his own terms. He wanted to remain at home and die in our bedroom, surrounded by the things he loved, holding my hand. That's a goal we achieved; he died peacefully, holding my hand at 4:05 p.m. on August 22, 1990.

Earlier that day, Paul and my mother talked by telephone. She told him she loved him, wished him a safe journey and asked him to give my Dad a hug from her when he got where he was going (my Dad had died two years earlier). He agreed. He and I also had a pact that when he got settled in, he would send a message letting me know he was safe.

As soon as Paul died, I called to tell my mother. Fr. Gary and I washed his body and called the funeral home. Shortly after Paul's body was taken from the house, Fr. Gary and I were sitting in our room talking. The smoke alarm went off for no apparent reason. It

continued

was just an odd event until several hours later when I
called my mother again, and she opened the
conversation by saying, "The strangest thing
happened just after you called. I was sitting in the
living room thinking about Paul and your Dad when
my smoke alarm went off . . ."

Paul's worst fear was that he would die and no
one would remember that he had lived. For that
reason the NAMES Project was very important to him.
He designed the panel himself and asked my mother
to help him make it. My mother lives in Florida so it
was a challenge to work on it together with 3,000
miles separating us. We managed, though, with love
and commitment. Paul loved flowers and irises were
his favorite. The bunnies represent us; the butterflies,
the freedom of his soul; and the epigraph is a variation
of the inscription found on my grandmother's and
father's tombstones.

He was the great love of my life; he'll live in my
heart forever and in the flowering plum and Japanese
maple tree that will be planted in his honor next
spring.

Michaele Wilk Houston

This quilt is actually a partner unfortunately to the one that was done in September 1987. Each heart holds the name of a person who we cared for regardless of race, creed, color, country of origin, occupation or status. They were ex-convicts, designers, musicians, physicians, the homeless. Each one was cared for and loved individually and given respect and dignity till the day they died.

Each one in their own special way has touched us and taught us, and although this is a tribute to their memory and their bravery, it has also been for us somewhat of a working-through some of the pain, as one can see the numbers are staggering.

A happy day for me will be when I can make a 3' × 6' panel that is blank.

I started making a banner for my friend Robin Hood (his real name) what seems a long time ago—in 1989. Before it was finished, his lover Earl Hambleton died and my project turned into a memorial for both of them.

Robin and Earl were very dear people to me and so very happy together that I wanted to ask the NAMES Project to sew their banners together on the Quilt to honor their bond of love. These banners are my way of saying hello and goodbye and perhaps thank you for being part of my life.

These lives were important to me, so in some manner I needed to reach out and do something for them and myself.

Robin taught me so many ways of having fun and laughing, and Earl was his more serious, organized counterpart. Together they were a wonderful mix of fun and serenity. Robin and Earl loved making a home together, the pleasures of gardening, playing with the dog, and cooking feasts were enough. Robin was a physical comedian, juggler, and acrobat who loved to gossip, had dreams of great success and always jested with everyone. Earl was also a dreamer (always of a better, more secure, and more secluded life) but was rooted in the high-tech world of lasers and Silicon Valley. I met Robin when working for the Pickle Family Circus in San Francisco. He was a performer and I was a technician. We found we had kindred spirits and spent much of our time backstage and on the road together. He always encouraged me to learn tricks and performance skills, and I in return tried to help with his creative projects, play bad music with him, or just lend an ear to his gossip and fantasies. We enjoyed getting crazy, as fun was at a premium in the Circus, and we also had our fights (Robin being terribly petulant and nasty and me being stubborn and unforgiving). Through all of this, our friendship prevailed and we became very close in a short time.

When Robin met Earl, he found an anchor for his wayward performer's life and after a few false starts they knew they were in love and became a happy couple, lucky to find joy in each other after years of detached experiences. As for Earl, I believe Robin was that necessary spark to his otherwise dull 9–5 life in a high-tech nonentity corporate world. They were well-matched and their relationship was healthy. It was this strength that brought them to their final days even more in love than they'd ever imagined. This is basically how I remember these two people, and I carry their banners in my heart always. I appreciated this project, as it helps give a physical and visual relationship to these feelings. I thank the NAMES Project for providing a way for me and others to express the feelings of loss and provide a means for our love to endure.

Carlos Hay Uribe

May 1, 1991

Today was her 29th birthday. But surely, this was a strange place for such an occasion; surely, this was not the usual way in which to celebrate 29 years of life!

People reminisced and spoke of her life. It hadn't been an easy one! She had brushes with the law, and that had complicated things. She had family and friends, but she had carved and followed her own route. She had a lengthy relationship with heroin, and that had said it all. Or so it had once seemed.

I sat in the subdued lighting and gazed at the simple, grey doeskin box and at the stilled and shrunken form beneath the glass slab. She once had been so attractive. Even in the hospital, the warmth of her person and the allure of her humor had been so clear.

I remembered that first visit, and then I remembered, even more clearly, my own apprehensions and uneasiness before that. After all, what did I know about drug addicts? Didn't they all suffer from some form or other of mental illness? Didn't their reputation alone make them people you wouldn't want to associate with? What was I, a street-ignorant, white, well-intentioned volunteer, going to do with/for this drug addict? Maybe it was all a mistake, a farfetched challenge, a bit of well-meant kindness that now had gotten out of hand!

I remembered her soft-spoken words, repeated

many times, "I'm in God's hands now." I could almost
see those gleeful eyes as I showed her the sketch I had
done of her. I could almost hear her embarrassed
appraisal of her own deteriorating looks.

How well I remember the day we met. As usual, I
was briefed beforehand. Part of this briefing included
phrases such as, "really nice person," "easy to talk
to" and "needs a friend." It also included phrases like
"black woman," "former prostitute," "jailed a few
times," "I.V. drug user" and "no real support
systems." The latter list stuck out in my mind. I had
visions of the women who work Howe Street. Women
who were desperate. Women who were willing to do
anything for a fix. Women who talked tough and acted
tough. Women with no real friends or family or
support systems due to years of lying and thieving.

All these thoughts raced through my mind as I
braced myself, took a deep breath, and walked into
her hospital room. I introduced myself. In a whispery
and gentle voice she said hello. Her face was gaunt
and her body scarred. Nevertheless, she was still one
of the most beautiful women I'd ever seen.

I stayed for about an hour that first day. When I
left the room I was reeling. She wasn't supposed to be
beautiful. She wasn't supposed to be kind, or have
feelings, or warmth or any of those kind of things. She
wasn't even supposed to be likable.

continued

A Client

That was July 22, 1986. On September 6, 1986, her 29th birthday, we buried her. I can't begin to tell you all that happened in those short weeks. Everything was in high gear and moving very fast. There was happiness and sadness and growth and love. There were a multitude of emotional turbulences that even now I haven't quite sorted out. I don't know if I ever will.

Like most people, I.V. drug abusers are a mixture of many things. And like most, they laugh, they cry, they love, they hurt, they live, they are human. They can raise kids. They can hold jobs. They can even be beautiful . . .

My client was no saint. She had good days, she had bad days. Some of her stories would make your hair curl. The point is that underneath her slavery to drugs was a human being. No better or worse than you or I. She just made some bad decisions and a few wrong turns . . . unfortunately hers killed her.

J. Timothy Oliver

Joe was a very close and dear friend; ex-roommate and fellow PWA. He was someone who meant a lot to me, and was always ready to listen to *all* I had to say. He was very caring and extremely concerned about AIDS and the impact it had on all affected . . .

I went to the theater with him to see "Beaches," starring Bette Midler; and will always be partial to the song she sang at the end of the movie, entitled "The Wind Beneath My Wings" (hence the theme of this panel).

Joe and I held hands and cried throughout the entire song about friendship, and I can still feel his hand squeezing mine every time I hear that song . . .

Lee Duplaa

Paul was my friend, lover and partner in life for 27 years. He passed away on February 16, 1989. Paul was an extraordinary man whose life was filled with many interests, a lifelong scholar, a highly regarded educator, a kind, caring and gentle man.

Due to our circumstances of family, jobs and community and also by our choice, our relationship was, for the most part, a closeted one. Perhaps the secrecy of our relationship is what made it so intense for all these years and made it so difficult to endure the shattering of that world, our life together.

My memories of Paul are many, but what I miss the most is not being able to talk to him, you know, those seemingly insignificant conversations: How was your day? Do you like my haircut? Let's go for a drive . . . Those little moments and things that are now even more cherished.

It was Paul's wish that the cause of his death not be revealed. Of course there were remarks, whispers and telling glances, and what we thought was our secret life; was not. It is amazing how death has a way of silencing and distancing people. Ironically, support and expressions of caring and love come from persons I least expected it from, and your family IS, no matter what.

In Paul's panel I have tried to illuminate his life, our relationship, and create a monument without revealing all . . . In fabric, I wanted the look of stone, monochromatic, symbolizing the secrecy of our life together and perhaps to make people take a closer look. The quote, "nothing of love is ever lost," is from a poem by a longtime friend of Paul, and something that I find comforting and most wholeheartedly believe in. The word VINCES with three crosses following, I found written in his daily diary, gaining frequency and fervor over the last months. It is a prayer: Vinces—you will overcome . . .

Although the making of this panel is born out of great sadness, it brings joy in helping to memorialize someone you love. Hopefully the panels, the Quilt, will enlighten the world that we are being left with unfillable voids in our lives and the world is less bright because of it.

Anthony

My friend Kevin died two days after his 29th birthday. He had been at the hospital for two weeks, with what I thought was only pneumonia. I never saw him during those two weeks. To this day I regret that. But over the phone, he kept telling me he'd be getting out soon. He did get out, but not in the way I had thought.

Two years have passed since then. Not a day goes by that I don't think "Kevin should be here." All the talks we had about what was to come of our lives in the days to come . . . It feels odd living out my ambitions, knowing Kevin's will only remain in the memories of those who knew him.

When I learned of the NAMES Project, I knew I had to make a panel for Kevin. While trying to think of what it was to be, I heard the song "Empty Chairs at Empty Tables," from the cast album of "Les Miserables." I knew then that was to become his panel. It expressed my feelings about Kevin being gone.

In the play, a man returns to the local tavern, where days earlier, all his friends were gathered, toasting to good times, sharing laughter, companionship and conversation. Now the man is

continued

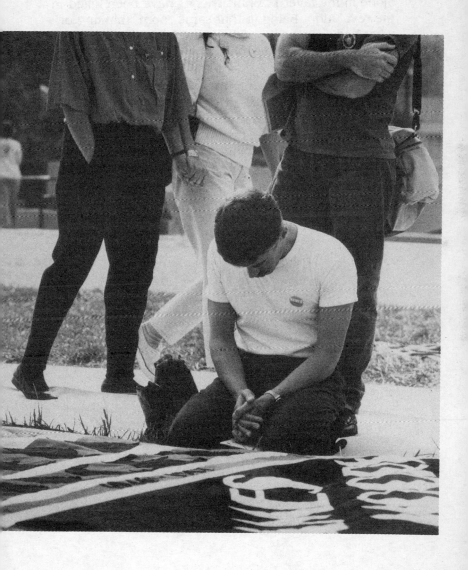

alone in the tavern. All his friends have been killed in the revolution. Being in that same room, thinking of what had once been, and realizing that those friends are all now gone. They should still be there, but are not.

This is what I feel with Kevin. He should be here. Kevin's panel illustrates a place once filled with life and happiness when he was there. Although he no longer sits at the table, his presence is still felt. But it's not the same as him being here. Kevin should be sitting at the table.

With love,

Tom Lawson

Remembering Raymond is difficult because both his life and death were difficult. Long before AIDS struck, Raymond faced formidable challenges. Family situations were strained so much that despite two brothers, a sister and a mother living nearby, Raymond died virtually alone. I suspect, though I will never know, that things were always this way: that Ray's family was never a source of support, that even when his brothers and sisters were in the same room, Raymond was nevertheless very much alone.

Part of this was due to Ray's personality. To say the least he was eccentric, shaped by fears and doubts and other withering winds for which psychologists have long, sterile labels: schizophrenia, hypochondria, paranoia. What he seemed to need most was someone to listen, to be patient, no matter how illogical or contradictory or even manipulative his words and behavior were. As far as I could tell, very few people did this for Ray. Recognizing his quirks, most of the people in his life, though they performed the motions of caring, kept Ray at a distance—and Ray could sense their indifference as surely as you or I can sense hot or cold.

No, Ray was alone in the world. As his Shanti volunteers, we tried to listen, and though I believe that we sometimes succeeded I know also that the task was often overwhelming.

. . . After all, isn't that what each of us wants? Not to be leveled into facelessness but to be treated as a unique, inimitable person? When we listened to Ray, we acknowledged his dignity. And when we listen to him now, in the silence of memory, we acknowledge it again.

Nobody had energy like David. He was a bright light. He bounded into our lives and left an indelible mark on all of those he touched. Impish, passionate, funny and with a grand sense of theatricality and style, David was 100 percent David at all times. He loved his mother and his family with the same fierce devotion he showed to his friends. David spent himself on others.

He loved to have lunch at Love's Barbeque in Hollywood and he loved Barbara Streisand and Barbara Cook and Sara Lee chocolate cakes and his slick black cat, Lady Luck . . .

He was Uncle David to my daughter and the children in our neighborhood and when times were hard, I remember him arriving on my daughter Jeanine's birthday with a beautiful dress for her from Saks Fifth Avenue. He cried out "Uncle David's here" and boy, was he! Almost immediately Barbara Streisand was blaring from my stereo and David was "holding court and giving high drama."

A lot of people depended on David. And a lot of people took advantage of him. I remember he read

Bette Davis's book and he used to quote it to me, saying "pity the strong." He said, "The weak people get all the empathy from others and all the support, but what about us? What about the strong ones?" David spent his life being strong for the rest of us. Even when he was very, very sick, it was difficult for him to tell us. He worried that his illness would upset us too much.

The last time I saw David, he was wearing a beautiful suit and carrying roses, gifts of course, and laughing out loud. He looked like a million bucks. He had come on a visit to San Francisco and that night we had a wonderful dinner together, along with David's friend Michael, and Paul who had driven in for the occasion. We laughed and remembered old times and we realized how those early experiences formed our lives as adults.

So many of us miss him so. I told him, shortly before he died, that we would all be together again in an instant, and I believe this is true. If there's anything about eternity that I look forward to, it is hearing David's voice calling out once again, "Uncle David's here!"

Susan E. Stauter

Phyllis Renee Wimberly was a resident of Jerusalem House in Atlanta, Georgia, where she lived her final days surrounded by friends and people who loved her very much. Phyllis died from AIDS at home, very peacefully. But she did not die alone, which was one of her biggest fears. Her friend and caregiver Martha Evans was with her . . .

The residents of Jerusalem House had planned a big Halloween party for late October. Phyllis's friend Martha Evans was making a pumpkin costume for Phyllis to wear. The last few days of her life, all Phyllis wanted was to be able to hold on until the party and wear her pumpkin. This was not to be.

We offer the pumpkin [on her quilt] as a symbol of the strength and courage with which Phyllis faced life and death.

Martha Evans

October 6, 1990

I had wanted to make this panel for my brother's ex-lover and best friend for a long time. I had the materials and design which my brother and I sent back and forth between Boston and New York City . . . but I never seemed to be able to start.

I went to see the Quilt here in Boston in June. It was overwhelming but so beautiful. It made me feel neglectful toward Bobby. I went home, and with my husband, stayed up until 3 a.m. working on the panel (Bobby . . . it made me miss you more).

Bobby, a native New Yorker, died last August. It's still hard to believe he's gone. Bobby with the sparkling blue eyes also wore a blue NYPD uniform, which he was very proud of. This is why we chose blue as our background. We also included symbols of his two loves: his Siamese cats and softball. Bobby was an umpire in the gay softball leagues.

Bobby was always a private person and it took a while for my brother to decide if Bobby would have wanted to be included in the Quilt. As Craig put it, "As soon as people realize that AIDS is not some dirty secret but a catastrophic problem that has been perpetuated by ignorance, we will all be better off . . . Bob would agree with that."

Please take good care of our memories, as I'm sure you will . . . If there is anything we can do to help, please let us know.

Thank you,
Diane C. Holmes

July 1988

KENNETH DAVID ADAMS

Kenneth David Adams was born May 6, 1956 in Dexter, MO . . . . Ken was not in good health from the day he was born, so that made him my "special" child, and a strong bond formed between us. He wanted to play the violin and even though we could not afford it, I purchased one for him. He learned to play beautifully. He developed a deep appreciation for classical music, loved good literature, liked to write stories.

As a teenager, Ken liked to sit up nights listening to Janis Joplin, Traffic, etc., with his step-brothers. He was more on the serious side than his brothers, but when he told a joke, it was even more funny for the fact that *he* was telling it . . .

As his mother, losing him, my special not-so-healthy but greatly gifted child, was and probably will be the hardest thing I have ever been through. Our bond was so strong he did not want to be in the hospital when the time came. He wanted to be at home with me, and I cared for him 11 months and sat with him through his last night.

Therapeutically working on Ken's AIDS quilt, my mind was flooded with loving memories of Ken's life. In recognition of those special memories, I have finished my degree in nursing. In caring for others, I can honor Ken's memory.

Betty Allen,
mother

April 1989

To be quite honest, I have no money. I am a college student in debt, and hardly making ends meet. So I cannot support this project financially.

I do, however, support the NAMES Project morally and spiritually. This notepaper may not be worth as much as currency to some, but I desperately hope that it is to you.

Please keep up the fight *against* AIDS and *for* the dignity of those who are victims.

Sincerely,

M.A. Stone

Dear Jim,

Thanks, buddy, for passing this way and touching my life. I'm a better man for having known you.

Thanks for your dry sense of humor, quietly stated. Thanks for your honesty and sensitivity. Thanks for your caring—for your family and friends, for wanting to "Save the Whales" and other creatures, and for history and your heritage.

Hollis and your sisters send their love.

Affectionately,

Dr. Lecil Hander

Bill was a college teacher, a North Beach bartender, and an art museum worker. In winter, he wore a purple and silver neck muffler. He loved Giotto's angels, their emotional contortions in the night sky.

Quite the romantic, Bill "loved to be in love," to quote from "The Rose." He luxuriated in the paradise of the world. During the rainy December that we first visited San Francisco, we stayed with friends across from the eucalyptus trees of Panhandle Park. Prisms of crystal hung in their windows. In the mornings, Noble played Mozart on his grand piano.

In the last three years of his life, Bill camped for days in Kauai's Waimea Canyon. I have pictures of him showering under a waterfall. After a long time of "just talking about it," he went to Ireland with his brother.

He kept telling me he was going to recuperate in the Canary Islands. During the final weeks of his illness, I picked up the phone to hear him chirping, "Tweet, tweet." It was hard to let go of that kind of spirit.

Lindell

My brother Jeff Reffitt died of AIDS on January 21, 1990. He was not only my brother, he was also my friend. Jeff lived his life the way he wanted, regardless of what society thought. He loved music and movies, dancing and being with his friends. It's too bad most of them deserted him when he needed them most.

Jeff had a witty, sometimes sarcastic, sense of humor. He was always concerned about whether his family would be OK after he was gone. We spent a lot of time with him in the three years before he died. Jeff, Mom, and I took several trips to various parts of Florida—Disney World, Key West, and Fort Lauderdale.

The panel that Mom and I made is done in the theme of Jeff's favorite movie, "The Wizard of Oz," and his favorite song, "Somewhere Over the Rainbow."

In the hospital in September of '89, he said to me, "I never thought I would hear myself say this, but, I will always be right here," and pointed to my heart. And that's where he remains with all of us.

I want Jeff to be remembered as someone who cared about other people—about the rights of other people—and was able to live his life the way that made him happy.

Jeff brought warmth, happiness, fun, and so much more into the lives of his family and friends. He is missed very deeply.

Beverly Parker and
Jana Schatzman

Dear NAMES Project,

Thank you for the chance to memorialize two people who meant a lot to me. Movies have always been at the center of my life, and the courage to come out of the closet came in no small part from validation in the works of these two men.

I am now heavily involved in GLAAD, because I know how much media images influence people's opinions.

You no doubt know who these men are, but just in case:

Vito Russo is a celebrated gay film critic and activist and the author of "The Celluloid Closet." It was my pleasure and honor to meet him last year, just seven months before he died of AIDS.

Bill Sherwood wrote and directed the film "Parting Glances."

Since both of these men were New Yorkers, I'd like these panels to be displayed in New York City. I'd also like them to return to Dallas, so I would see it. Beyond that, it's up to you.

Again, thanks.

Alonso Duralde

SCOTT LAGO ═══════════════════════

(From remarks made at Scott's memorial service in Atlanta, Georgia)

I loved Scott Lago very much. Many of you will have known him most of his life. I feel blessed to have been his friend for three years. They were very special ones.

In a sense, I knew Scott before I ever met him. Kyle Gibson, the "Nightline" producer, and I were screening Kyle's piece on the Quilt several days before the 1988 display in Washington, D.C. As Scott's face and voice came on the monitor, Kyle looked up and said, "That's Scott Lago—he's SO wise."

We met for the first time at the press conference several days later. I won't say that I saw the wise part of Scott immediately—the wisecrack part was more readily apparent.

But as we became better and better friends, the special qualities of wisdom and insight and sensitivity were the ones that I felt most honored to share.

And yes—we laughed and danced and sang and dished: the evenings with Linda and David at the Five Oaks, A Night of a Thousand Gowns, the night in San Francisco when we recast the Mary Tyler Moore show with staff members at the NAMES Project.

I will remember more, though, the thoughtful times: with Linda and Beth in Boston talking about our families, our hopes and dreams, or the night in Washington we stayed up all night plotting Scott's future, or in Austin, Texas, Scott sharing his concerns about staff members who were not able to experience the Quilt because of the press of work at home.

And there was one very special evening I want to share with you. Scott came from San Francisco for "Skating for Life," a DIFFA benefit with about 30 figure-skating stars from around the world. He had always loved watching Olympic and other skating programs on television, but had never seen a skating show live. Scott's wonder, his awe, his total pleasure at the beauty of seeing Scott Hamilton, Rosalynn Sumners, and others from a distance of five feet was extraordinary. I think that evening we felt as close emotionally and physically as we ever did.

There were many, many other occasions, many phone conversations, many shared secrets and emotions and simply fun times. I will always be grateful for having had such a wonderful friend.

AIDS is a dreadful disease, and a dreadful death. If Scott's personality and individuality, if his work with the NAMES Project AIDS Memorial Quilt has moved two people, or two hundred people, or two hundred thousand people to care about AIDS and to do something about it, he has contributed something extraordinary to this planet.

I loved Scott very much. I miss him mightily.

Nancy Blanford

August 5, 1991

Bruce Richard Taylor was born deaf in 1951 to a hearing family in Toledo, Ohio. Following the accepted medical advice of the day, Bruce was brought up to lip read and mainstreamed through public hearing schools to make him "normal" and to fit into a hearing world. Intelligent and with a winning personality, he smiled his way through high school without having his potential recognized or tapped.

Eighteen years old before he learned sign language and a form of communication that opened worlds for him, he never recovered from his loathing for a silent, boring school system.

Bruce grew to be a man of taste and charm with very decided opinions. When we met, it seemed everyone in New York knew Bruce and loved him. In 1984, he was elected Mr. ERAD (Empire Rainbow Alliance of the Deaf), a gay deaf organization in New York City. He attended the international convention in Toronto as their representative, and won the title of Mr. RAD, 1984. This was a personal triumph. The man glowed.

When he became ill, he lost the sight in his left eye. We were terrified that he would lose his vision completely. His good eye lasted as long as he did.

Bruce's divorced parents came to see him separately at first, but later together as a family. From my diary when Bruce's father first came to visit him from Michigan:

"As we were leaving the hospital tonight, Bruce walked us to the elevator. He was upset. Finally, he told me he had noticed a lot of activity in the room next door. Nurses running. He came out into the hall and saw a young man crying. His friend had just died. Bruce asked him, "AIDS?" The man nodded. Bruce said, "Me, too." They both cried and hugged each other. Bruce's father said, "What did he say?"

Bruce taught me to communicate and that communication can take many forms, but that the lack of communication is a silent vacuum. The manual symbol on Bruce's banner of a raised hand with three digits extended is the American Sign Language ideogram for the phrase, "I love you."

Bruce, I love you.

Thomas Slack and Jon Rager

P.S.: Jon Rager died of AIDS on April 17, 1990. Quilt panels have been made in his memory.

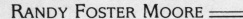

One might note that Randy's memorial service was held on August 22, 1987—his birthday. Instead of a closing hymn, we were asked to sing "Happy Birthday." Very few could find their voice.

James G. Finch

This quilt has been made in memory of my brother, Leonard. Leonard can be remembered as someone who, when healthy, had boundless energy for enjoying life—which he did much of the time. His spirit was young and stayed young with a twinkle of hope down to the very last moment . . .

Leonard loved in his own way and did the things that he wished to do. I am glad he'd made those choices early on, because he didn't have time to waste.

Leonard loved New York City, he loved the night, loved to dance right through the night, loved dining alone in his pink and purple apartment, loved to make a fashion statement, and later came to love the feeling of being with family, of having a home with us and of each day that he was alive.

We all contributed a part to the quilt and listened to many of Leonard's dance tapes as we put the quilt together.

I'd love one last dance with my brother.

Susan Sprung

To the entire staff of the NAMES Project, my heartfelt thanks for making the Quilt possible. The weekend of June 3–5 was one of the most memorable weekends I have ever experienced. Even when I was not monitoring on the Quilt, I could not bear being away from it.

When I was in D.C. last October, I purposely stayed away from it, since Tommy had just died on September 28, and I did not know if I could deal with it. He was, and always will be, my closest friend. His loss to me was overwhelming. Although we were just friends, we were as close to each other, if not closer, than lovers. We cried and laughed our way through life. On my 50th birthday he teased me about my having to attend his 50th in a wheelchair since he always referred to me as his much older sister. We played together in life and we worked together in life strengthening the gay community of Cleveland. We served as board members of our organization, of which I still serve as a tribute to him. He organized the gay softball league here in Cleveland, and that is what his panel is all about, the patches reflecting the teams Number 7 played on.

He was the one who made me sponsor a team called Mitzi's, which he personally led to a championship. Tomboys was his team, which he sponsored after his diagnosis. Although they never won a game, he was a winner while his frail body would give it its all. Even in his last hours, his final gesture to me was a "high five."

Knowing Tommy the way I did, and the way he joined everything in sight, I know he would want to be part of the NAMES Project. In making his panel, I, too, received so much satisfaction. In his jean pockets are personal messages that we put in as our final farewell. The panel did get wet with tears, yet the laughs were there when I remembered the crazy situations we would get into. I know he wanted to go to D.C. last year, but thanks to you guys, he will be able to join me this October.

I don't know if you can imagine how much I appreciate everything you guys have done for thousands like me. Thank you ever so much, and if I can be of any assistance to you, let me know . . . I know Tommy thanks you for letting him, the political activist that he was, be in Washington.

With sincere thanks,

Gene Witts, President,
Northern Ohio Coalition

The last image we have of David is when he left for Amsterdam in December 1983. We had fixed him a huge picnic basket of wine and cheese to travel on the plane with, and he later said he had to pig out on the whole basket before they would let him board the plane.

Although we talked to him long distance and on holidays and special occasions many times, we never knew of his illness or suffering until after his death. We missed him terribly after he moved from Houston, but we could always confirm our friendship by phone.

Now, we cherish having known his gentle nature and good humor, rather than regret his passing.

Thank you, David.

Love,

Don Robinson and
Doug Scott

As the panel indicates, Tom Smith loved movies. As a child he spent many a Sunday afternoon at the movies with his grandmother and brother and the scarier the movie, the better. The drive-in was our favorite. Load up the car with goodies and off we'd go. As a teen, he never missed the new movie out and would come home and tell me all about it . . .

Tom went off on his own adventure, leaving Mentor at the age of 19 for San Francisco. I cried, and he told me not to cry because now I would have a place to visit. And visit him I did, and we went to Chinatown, Fisherman's Wharf, the Golden Gate Bridge, beautiful churches, great restaurants, and, of course, we went to the movies.

I missed Tom but we had long talks on the phone and he soon became not only my son, but my best friend . . .

I love and miss Tom so much. Twenty-seven years old is too young to die. There should have been a lot more movies for Tom to see here. I'm sure that Tom is in a far better place watching great movies and one day we'll be watching them together again.

Judy
(Tom Smith's mother)

JED

I finished sewing Jed's panel before Christmas. It was a difficult, but comforting task. And I've been putting off writing this eulogy or description or essay and sending it to you. I guess I don't want to say goodbye or put this ending of sorts on my grieving.

But I really won't ever completely say goodbye to Jed; I have so many memories. So many things I own were given to me by Jed. Little funny things, that are now even more precious. Last week, I was packing to move and I came across so much: the sparkly gold socks he got for me at a Goodwill store to go with my gold lamé tennis shoes; a "Campfire Marshmallow" tin; postcards from all over the West; a red corduroy shirt.

Jed and I were best friends for quite some time. Practically inseparable. We went to graduate school together at the University of Idaho (the gold and silver trim on his panel reflect the school's colors) . . . We took naps together, mowed lawns together, and shared many hangovers together. You see, Jed and I both drank a lot (that's an understatement). But we were much more than just drinking buddies. Our friendship survived my sobering up and joining A.A. He never got to.

I know so many details about him, so many of his foibles and quirks. Remembering them saddens me the most, but keeps Jed very close and dear to me. He drank his coffee black and in small mugs so he could drink it all before it got cold. He smoked Vantage cigarettes except when he had coupons to try others for less. He would reuse postage stamps from letters where the cancellation marks missed the stamps. He named his car "Rusty." He liked the dark meat of the chicken best. He tried to tame the wild cats and kittens at his dad's place. He invented the magic and joy of "found objects"—objects one finds on sidewalks, like lost earrings, single gloves, that sort of thing. I still collect "found objects." . . .

I last saw Jed when he came to Washington for the Gay Rights March last October . . . We spent an afternoon together and then "did lunch" the following day. He seemed calmer and more confident than I had known him to be.

On November 16, I got the phone call from a friend of his. Jed had committed suicide sometime the week before. He sent notes to a few people on November 9th and his body was found November 14th. He used carbon monoxide poisoning in his car parked in the cemetery of his hometown. A few years earlier, he had shown me the place and had told me that when his "life got to be too much" that this was where he would kill himself. (I am oddly comforted by knowing where he died.)

I found out that Jed was diagnosed with AIDS sometime last summer. He may have made his decision then. It seems that by having AIDS, Jed's "life got to be too much" . . .

Thank you for giving me a way to grieve—in a way that is healing and, God willing, helpful in ending this horrible disease.

Martha Frederick

March 1, 1988

Before my brother Ron died of AIDS, I promised him that I would create a panel for the Quilt in his memory, for I knew how important it was to him. He was pleased, since he had done the same for his lover, Ken Wilkes, only three years before. Ken was the love of his life, and tragically, they were only together for a very short time before Ken discovered he had AIDS. Ken died 18 months after being diagnosed.

During the last month of Ron's illness, I spent a great deal of time with him in his apartment. His bed had been moved into the living room where he had a wonderful view of the San Francisco skyline, the city he loved so much. Ron also loved anything Italian, the opera and theatre, the arts and traveling. He was extremely meticulous, an avid reader, and a great cook. He was a kind, good person, particularly close to our parents, the wonderful people of Trinity Episcopal Church, and the Crisio Group he led. He had tremendous faith in God and was an inspiration to me.

Trying to decide what to put on Ron's panel came easily. Ron had a favorite print hanging in his living room of a "de colores" cross that had been done by Ken. I decided to try to recreate this cross, using it as the focal point on the panel. The purple cloth covered his ashes at the memorial service. I had discovered the note to Ron from God on his bulletin board after his death. Aside from the fact that it was a beautiful note and another example of his faith in God, it also gave me the opportunity to preserve his handwriting, which I had always admired.

I thank you wonderful people at the NAMES Project for giving so many relatives and friends the opportunity to remember their loved ones in such a beautiful and meaningful way.

Betty Pellizzer

March 1990

Mark at age 37 was a victim of AIDS.

We met Mark in 1984 over the phone. Mark and our son Bill were lovers . . . We are most proud of our son Bill and the love and care he gave Mark. We are also happy we had the opportunity to get to know this young man . . .

Let us hope that this great NAMES Project will make our government and the population of this wonderful country of ours aware of the great need to end the slaughter of men, women and children through finding a way to stop AIDS. We want it for all, and yes, selfishly, for our son Bill.

Loving parents,
Jeanne and Chuck

In October of 1990, I was among the many people who visited the Quilt in Los Angeles. I don't know what I was expecting when I entered that church, but when I exited, my views on AIDS and its sufferers were completely changed.

Although I was aware of AIDS and the statistics broadcast on the news, viewing the Quilt shocked me into dealing with those numbers on a more personal level. I was overwhelmed with emotion as I viewed each panel. To think of each panel as a representation of other human beings, their lives cut short by a vicious disease, forced me to realize the true tragedy of this crisis.

Even though it has been over five months since I visited the Quilt, I think about that experience often. It is these thoughts that have prompted me to write to you. I have also taken some time today to write to the President, to express my outrage due to the lack of funds being provided for AIDS research and treatment.

It is impossible to adequately express my gratitude to you and the many people who worked so hard to bring the Quilt to the general public. Due to your efforts, I was able to gain the knowledge and understanding necessary to recognize that AIDS is a human issue of monumental proportion. Thank you again for all of your hard work.

Sincerely,

Gayle J. Crockett

March 19, 1991

Tim was a simple, sensitive, timid young man, who cared for and loved in a way which many never understood.

As a child his family life was difficult. He was raised by a hard-working mother abandoned by her husband at an early age.

He was raised a Catholic, and taught that to love another man was a sin.

His family was part American Indian, and as such there were lots of relatives, lots of strong family ties through them that he didn't have in his home.

I think that ours was his first real home, and I the first strong dependable loving man in his life. Tim often spoke of his envy for the home I was raised in and the obvious love of our family for each other and for him.

In the early stages of our relationship, before I really understood this incredible man, I questioned his love, because he rarely used the word "LOVE" and it was always so easy for me. In the summer of 1985, his mother visited us in our home in Boston. The day Tim's mom left, Tim told me that she told him how very much she loved him, and that she had never told him that before in his entire life. I then understood.

Tim and I met a young man at the Deaconness Hospital in Boston . . . The Kaposi's and other ailments that this young man had were so awful that it was not until weeks later that I found out this was our friend

Ted. I had spoken to Ted while he was receiving a chemo treatment next to Tim. Tim didn't speak a word. When Ted left, Tim began to cry because he wanted so much to reach out and help Ted, but he couldn't speak the words.

Tim bought a beautiful book of photos of Boston, and wrapped it and brought it to the hospital to pass along, still not knowing this was our friend Ted. A few weeks later we saw Ted and his mom at the hospital. Ted was so elated by the gift from Tim, even more so when he realized we had not recognized him. Ted realized that Tim's gift was from his heart, not from a feeling of obligation to a friend.

Tim spoke his love and caring, again, without words.

On his last visit to the hospital, before going home to die in his own home, in my arms, Tim verbalized all he had never been able to before. Tim talked comfortably about his love and about all the ways in which he always showed his love rather than spoke of it. I realized for the first time that words mean so little, and that it takes action to communicate real love . . .

A room has been dedicated, by family and friends, in Tim's name at the Gay and Lesbian Counseling Center. Tim's room is dedicated to support groups for persons dealing with the anxieties associated with the AIDS virus.

Frank Ribaudo

... We didn't have much time to create a panel ... with the help of Peter's aunts, uncle and cousins, we tried to create a panel that would typify Peter.

I do hope your project makes our government realize how many great individuals we are losing to this disease and to put more money toward finding a way to stop it.

Sincerely,

D. Gordon and
Luella W. Hollinger

September 3, 1987

Dear Mr. President,

I am writing to you today to express my outrage—
my disbelief—my anger—my sadness because of the
complete silence from you concerning the beautiful
NAMES Project Quilt that was on the Ellipse directly in
front of your house last weekend . . .

The Quilt has come to Washington D.C. for three
years in a row. For those three years, there has been
silence from the White House . . . I keep asking, *Why*?
WHY?

The Quilt is such a beautiful and loving thing. It
shows that people affected by this disease are kind
and gentle people. It shows names and lives behind
the cold, hard statistics. I could go on and on about
this . . .

What I really want to ask you is "Why the
silence?" I would like to know why you can't say the
word AIDS publicly . . . Mr. President, please do not
remain silent. Lead this country in the education and
fight against this crisis. You are leading the country for
the fight against drugs, please lead the country and the
world in the fight against AIDS.

Did you know that this year [1989] was the last
year that the Quilt would ever be shown in its
entirety? After this year, the Quilt will be too large to
show in one place . . . The Quilt will be back in
Washington each and every year in some form until

continued

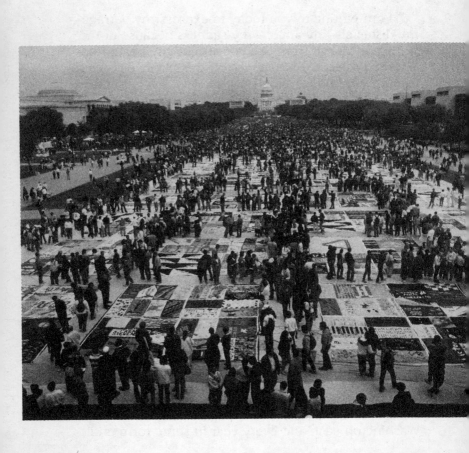

this AIDS epidemic is over. We will not remain silent.
We can no longer accept your silence. You, along with
everyone on this earth, will eventually become
affected personally somehow by this terrible
disease . . .

Thank you for listening to me, and I pray you will
find kindness and gentleness in your heart to act
NOW.

Sincerely,

James D. Migliore

I would like to briefly share with you my experience of this past Saturday evening.

I had been working very hard and long hours, and decided to take a walk up Market Street. As I approached Castro Street, I found the NAMES Project open, with two people sewing. I went in, as I had not visited since last Christmas. A woman sewing greeted me and encouraged me to look around.

When I went to the back of the room, I saw one quilt section hanging . . . it featured three quilts made by family and friends of Lou Scavarda, a wonderful friend who died in 1988.

Lou's death was a sad and difficult time for me. I knew we had some unfinished business, and I understood that I was intuitively directed to go into the shop. It was a very touching few moments. I needed to say "Hello, Lou," and goodbye again.

I recalled that when the NAMES Project first opened, Lou and I volunteered numerous times to cut 3' × 6' material segments. The work was rather mindless, but its purpose very emotional. It didn't occur to me then that the quilt would have the impact it has had on me since Lou's death.

Thank you for having the shop open. Thank you to the woman encouraging me to look further.

I hope the enclosed check helps you and others to keep the message, and ultimately people, alive.

Alan Hayes

October 4, 1991

I am so happy about the Quilt going back to Washington. I am on a fixed income—is there some way ones like me could be helped out with the cost of the trip? As I get Social Security, disability, and SSI ($650 a month), this means so much to me. Ron McKay, my friend and lover, just died April 8, 1991. Maybe I can help in the office doing something.

Thank you,

Raymond H. Clark

I am interested in adding a panel to the Quilt . . .

I was fortunate to see the Quilt displayed this past fall in Washington, D.C. with my brother. It was a very emotional time [as] *together* we smiled, cried, and held each other as we walked down the aisles. What a beautiful memory to have shared with him, but an ugly nightmare of a disease.

I recently lost my brother to AIDS (in February 1990). I'm trying to realize I can't have him back or see him again, but through the panel, he will always remain on earth. I miss him terribly and need to make my hands busy. I teach 21 preschoolers, but I need to use my creativity as my brother would have.

I am so thankful that you are there for us.

Jamie Miller and
Jon C. Nathanson

On October 24, 1989, I lost someone who was very, very special to me. His name was Joe Grassi.

Joey was more to me than just my brother, he was my best friend.

Joey and I were never embarrassed by the fact that he had AIDS. There was no reason to be. It's not a disgrace, it's not a punishment from God. It's a disease that any one of us can get . . .

It hurt me more than anything in this world to watch him fade from a big, strong, healthy man to a blind, frail, very sick, thin man. I would have given up anything in my life to make him well again.

Having a panel added to the Quilt is now my biggest dream, but I am by no means a seamstress. I was wondering if there is anyone who can help me make a panel in his honor . . . I am even willing to come to the workshop on my vacation from work to have this dream come true.

If any of you had known him, I'm sure a hundred of you would be knocking on my door to sit and help me with the work . . .

Yours truly,

Patty Mosqueda

January 19, 1990

Dear Gepetto,

It has been almost four months since I met you at the Bakersfield College Quilt display. My daughter, son and I presented my brother's quilt to you. That was such a beautiful and special ceremony. I will always remember that weekend . . .

I think that the work that you are doing for the NAMES Project is magical . . . You are a loving person and have helped me through a difficult period. Thank you, and I hope we meet again.

When I presented Dante's quilt, it did not have a hem or a descriptive letter about him. It's been hard emotionally to sit down and write. It seems easier not to deal with issues that are painful.

The quilt was presented on Saturday and I stayed up all of the previous night making the quilt. I knew that the quilt would be accepted even if it didn't have a hem . . . I hope that the good people at the NAMES Project were able to complete it for me.

I was told that the quilt would be assigned a number. I'm not sure how to go about obtaining that number. I was hoping that you might be able to get that information for me. I would like to pass it on to friends and family, so that they will be able to see the Quilt in their cities . . .

Your friend,
Colleen Sandberg

This check is in memory of my friend Mark Tsakirgis, whom I loved dearly. I did not get a chance to say goodbye to Mark as he only told me he had AIDS a few weeks before he died. Also, he did not mix his "two" lives.

I would love to know who made his quilt—it was beautiful . . . The Quilt helped me to say my goodbyes.

God bless you,

Beth Leney

July 21, 1988

My wife and I recently attended the Sixth International AIDS Conference at San Francisco's Moscone Civic Center. While we found the scientific presentations extremely interesting, the highlight of the week for us was our visit to the AIDS Memorial Quilt displayed at Fort Mason Center . . . We had never seen the Quilt before. We could not help but contrast the sad, quiet (and haunting) peace of Fort Mason with the loud, blaring activity in and around Moscone.

While visiting the Quilt, we had a small sense of the sadness and ultimate rage that must have been produced in those persons afflicted with the disease. We also realized that a number of the activists both taking part in the conference and protesting outside were also afflicted. It became very clear to us that the noise that drowned out Secretary Sullivan's closing speech was a reflection of that rage, an emotion which even the most well-meaning scientists might not understand . . . no matter how much they studied AIDS in their laboratories . . .

. . . Thanks to the Quilt and all those panels for helping us not to forget, even for a moment, the destruction of AIDS.

Sincerely,

Joseph N. Vitale and
Theresa Z. O'Connor

July 11, 1990

We are 15 years old and live in Florida. After seeing the AIDS Quilt at the University of Montana on August 12, 1990, we were wondering what we can to do to help educate people, and help them see and feel the things we felt!

We aren't exactly sure how we can help, but we feel we need to do something . . .

Thank you!

Sincerely,

Robyn L. Moorman and
Shannon M. Lapinsky

August 15, 1990

Thank you for sharing the Quilt with America. Seeing the Quilt in Washington, D.C. with my family was a profoundly moving experience. It changed us all for the better.

I must admit that prior to seeing the Quilt, my experience of the gay community was limited to childish gawking while passing through the gay areas of our major cities. My view of "them" was negative simply because "they" were so "different."

Then, last month, my wife, my two 12-year-old children, and I were visiting Washington, D.C. when we stumbled upon the Quilt displayed near the White House.

We were fascinated. We walked in and around this vast, colorful welcome mat of memories— welcome because it, and the people there, bid us welcome. We walked in and around the friends, lovers, and family members of those who have so tragically succumbed to this wretched disease in the prime of their lives.

The grief, the love, the loss and the hope of those present was palpable and powerful. We felt the emotion, as if those remembered were our own. The Quilt may represent the world of people with AIDS. Yet it is our world, too . . .

I am so very glad my children experienced this moment at an early age. They shared in our emotional rescue from intolerance. They tell me that in school, gays and others who are "different" are ridiculed. I hope that my children will appreciate their new-found tolerance as they mature . . .

Please accept my thanks to you and the families, friends and volunteers who are the NAMES Project for allowing us to share in your love, in your pain, and your tolerance. Please continue to show the Quilt so that others may have their tolerance levels challenged, and changed, as we did.

Sincerely,

Richard J. Simonsen
Professor, School of Dentistry,
University of Tennessee,
Memphis

... It's this aspect of the Quilt—as a symbol of communal strength—that inspires me to continue supporting it. Too many others face the day when they, too, will need to draw from that well of strength, and I want the Quilt to be there for them just as it was for me.

Mike's panel—my panel—is now surrounded by scores more, and has traveled the nation on a truly historic journey. Tens of thousands of people have seen it and been moved by it.

Over half a million dollars have been raised because of the tour, allowing people with AIDS a measure of hope and dignity by giving them access to vital, social, medical and legal services.

It amazes me that something as simple and time-honored as a Quilt could do all that. But it also reassures me to know, amidst this harrowing crisis, maddening politicking, and mysterious researching, that it is humanity that guides us through this epidemic. And what better symbol of humanity, American style, than a Quilt? ...

We all must continue to be as generous to the Quilt as it has been to us. I know I will continue to do everything I can to see that the Quilt remains a living symbol of hope and love for as long as the epidemic afflicts us.

Sincerely,

Sue Caves

October 1988

I am currently a student at Rutgers University . . . Fortunately, a friend and I took the time to view the Quilt last spring. We left with eyes filled with tears and walked home in silence that day. We will never forget the emotional impact the Quilt had on us.

Since we both have not been directly affected by AIDS in that we do not know anyone personally who has it or has died from it, the Quilt took on a special meaning for us. It showed us the *reality* of AIDS. This is something that is difficult to manifest to undergraduate college students. But the Quilt did it. It is so important to many people in so many different ways.

Because I am paying for my education I am unable to send you a donation more sufficient. I would just like to thank everyone for contributing to such a great cause. I would also like to volunteer some of my own time, but am not sure whom to get in touch with . . .

God Bless!

Terry Ryan

January 7, 1991

DAVID HOLMES, JR. ═══════════

Dear NAMES Project:

I get so many requests for money in the mail that I was ready to throw this one away, too, until I read it.

I have seen the Quilt in its entirety each time it has come to Washington, and have watched the panels of people I know unfold each time. As a member of the gay community and a dancer, I have watched too many people get sick and die.

My close friend and teacher, David Holmes, Jr., died almost a year ago. I have thought about him every day since then. His memory remains alive for many of us. His life was lived with joy, and that is still his gift to us.

This contribution is to keep other people's memories alive, and to remind the world that each person who had died of AIDS was a loved individual.

When will the tears stop?

Donna Coupard

January 8, 1991

This panel was made in memory of my brother's friend, Alan Thompson. Alan passed away from AIDS in February of 1985; the day my brother, Tim Eyler, was diagnosed. Tim and Alan loved each other very much, so I hope this will serve as a tribute to that love.

Alan was from a well-to-do family in North Carolina. When he told them he was gay, he was disowned by his family except his mother. She was a wonderful, compassionate woman who always ended her letters and conversations with "Always remember," and Alan would reply, "Remember what?" To which she would answer, "I love you!"

Alan brought that special love into his relationship with Tim. That phrase, "Always remember," kept them going through the rough months of Alan's illness. Later, during Tim's illness, he and I used it as our own special way of showing our love for each other.

Alan passed away in February of 1985. Tim died 15 months later.

Susan Harrell

I am a freshman at Virginia Commonwealth University and yesterday, upon the persuasion of a good friend of mine, I decided to go see the AIDS Quilt exhibit. However, I wasn't prepared for it. I had never been so moved by an exhibit before. I read some of the things including a poem entitled, "I did not die," another poem comparing the colors blue, purple, and red to the AIDS victim David Razien, and a letter written by a boy named Chris to his parents. After looking, and reading, and feeling, I felt as though I had changed. I even cried.

I had always been brought up thinking that AIDS was a homosexual disease, or that heterosexuals got it by "sleeping around." I was raised to believe that gays were bad people not to be associated with. But not anymore. I read the booklets of information and was shocked by how wrong I was. And I realized that it doesn't matter if you're black, or white, a male or a female, or even a homosexual or a heterosexual, you're still a person. A person who has feelings, thoughts, who knows pain and joy. And that you have people, friends and family, that care about you and cry when you're gone. We're all the same. We can't just ostracize AIDS victims like ancient civilizations did to the lepers, because they need us, and in a way, we need them, too.

The last quilt had this logo on it:

$$\text{AIDS} - \cancel{\text{Ignorance}} = \heartsuit\,\text{Love \& Care}$$

I believe wholeheartedly in this because it happened to me and if it can happen to me, it can happen to anyone. Finally, I'd just like to say, thank you, for everything.

October 11, 1991

To me this panel signifies hope as well as loss.

"The Last One" refers to the final loss of individual life due to AIDS. He or she will mark the end of this devastating virus. When that person can be named we will begin to heal like we did as a nation for the Vietnam casualties.

I hope this quilt will find a permanent display and be preserved. Having been diagnosed, there will someday be a panel in my name. It's comforting to know it will be joined to the others and dearly remembered.

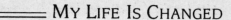

A student at San Luis Obispo High School, saw the Quilt in her school gymnasium, and left this simple note in response.

My life is changed.

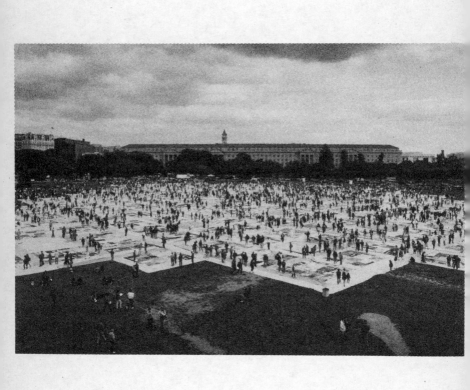

... I know that wherever the Quilt is displayed, all the beautiful souls represented on the Quilt are looking down from Heaven and smiling and comforting those of us left behind.

Thank you,

Jeanett Jay Kainer

How to Create a Panel ══════════

The memorial panels that make up the NAMES Project AIDS Memorial Quilt were made by all sorts of people, in all kinds of colors, fabrics, and styles. You do not have to be a professional artist to create a moving, personal tribute. It doesn't matter if you use paint or fine needlework; any remembrance is appropriate.

You may choose to create a panel privately, as a personal memorial to someone you've loved, but we encourage you to follow the traditions of old-fashioned sewing and quilting bees, and include your friends, family and coworkers.

1. *Design the panel.* Include the name of your friend or loved one. Feel free to include additional information, such as the dates of birth and death, and a home town. Please limit each memorial panel to one individual.

2. *Choose your materials.* Remember that the Quilt is folded and unfolded many times, so durability is crucial. A medium-weight, non-stretch fabric such as cotton works best. The *finished* panel must be 3 feet by 6 feet (90 cm × 180 cm), so when you cut the fabric leave an extra 2–3 inches on each side for a hem.

3. *To construct your panel, you might want to use some of the following techniques:*
Applique: Sew fabric letters and small mementos onto the background fabric. Please do not use glue; it will not last.

Paint: Brush on textile paint or color-fast dye, or use an indelible ink pen. No "puffy" paint, it is too sticky.
Stencil: Trace your design onto the fabric with a pencil, lift the stencil, then use a brush to apply textile paint.
Collage: A variety of materials can be added to the panel, but please make sure they won't tear the fabric (avoid glass and sequins for this reason) and please avoid very bulky objects. The best way to include photos or letters is to photocopy them onto iron-on transfers, iron them onto 100 percent cotton fabric and sew that fabric to the panel. You may also put the photo in clear plastic vinyl and sew it to the panel (off-center so it avoids the fold).

4. *When your panel is finished,* it must measure 3 feet by 6 feet (90 cm × 180 cm). If you can't hem it yourself, leave two or three inches on each side and we will hem it for you.

5. *Please take the time to write a one or two-page letter* about the person you've remembered. The letter might include your relationship to them, how he or she would like to be remembered and maybe a favorite memory. If you can, send us a photograph with the letter for our archives.

6. *Be sure to include the following information in your letter:* your name, address, phone number (and the names and addresses of others who may have helped make the panel), cities you would like to see your panel displayed in, your relationship to the

person you've made the panel for and the person's full name if it isn't on the panel (optional). Remember that once submitted, all panels become the sole property of the NAMES Project Foundation.

7. *If you can, please make a financial contribution to help pay* for the cost of adding your panel to the Quilt. The NAMES Project depends on the support of panel makers to help us preserve the Quilt and keep it on display. Gifts of $100 or more will be acknowledged in our annual FRIENDS OF THE QUILT donor roll as Panel Sponsors. Thank you.

Pack everything carefully, and send it to The NAMES Project Foundation, 2362 Market Street, San Francisco, California 94114. Or, for more information, you can phone us at (415) 863-5511.

LOVED ONES REMEMBERED